MEMORIES

OF A

CARIBOO DOCTOR

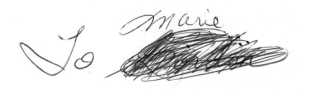

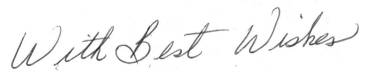

To Marie ~~~~~~

With Best Wishes

Len

By Len Maher, M.D.

Note for Librarians: A cataloguing record for this book is available from Library and Archives
Canada at www.collectionscanada.ca/amicus/index-e.html
ISBN 1-4120-5926-7

*Printed in Victoria, BC, Canada. Printed on paper with minimum 30% recycled fibre. Trafford's print shop
runs on "green energy" from solar, wind and other environmentally-friendly power sources.*

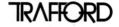

Offices in Canada, USA, Ireland and UK
This book was published *on-demand* in cooperation with Trafford Publishing. On-demand
publishing is a unique process and service of making a book available for retail sale to the
public taking advantage of on-demand manufacturing and Internet marketing. On-demand
publishing includes promotions, retail sales, manufacturing, order fulfilment, accounting and
collecting royalties on behalf of the author.

Book sales for North America and international:
Trafford Publishing, 6E–2333 Government St.,
Victoria, BC v8t 4p4 CANADA
phone 250 383 6864 (toll-free 1 888 232 4444)
fax 250 383 6804; email to orders@trafford.com
Book sales in Europe:
Trafford Publishing (uk) Ltd., Enterprise House, Wistaston Road Business Centre,
Wistaston Road, Crewe, Cheshire cw2 7rp UNITED KINGDOM
phone 01270 251 396 (local rate 0845 230 9601)
facsimile 01270 254 983; orders.uk@trafford.com
Order online at:
trafford.com/05-0827

10 9 8 7 6 5 4 3

CONTENTS

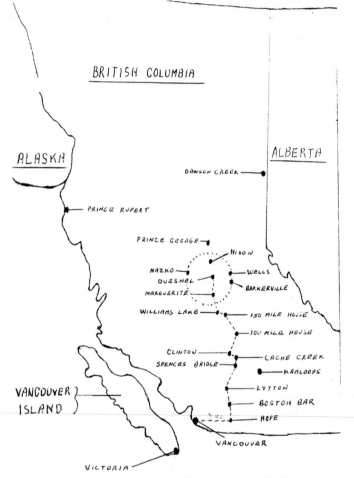

BRITISH COLUMBIA

ALASKA

ALBERTA

DAWSON CREEK

PRINCE RUPERT

PRINCE GEORGE

HIXON

NAZKO

WELLS

QUESNEL

MARGUERITE

BARKERVILLE

WILLIAMS LAKE — 150 MILE HOUSE

100 MILE HOUSE

CLINTON

SPENCES BRIDGE — CACHE CREEK

KAMLOOPS

LYTTON

BOSTON BAR

VANCOUVER
ISLAND

HOPE

VANCOUVER

VICTORIA

JOURNEY FROM VANCOUVER TO QUESNEL - JULY, 1951 _ _ _ _ _ _
AREA SERVICED BY QUESNEL HOSPITAL AND DOCTORS.......

i

ACKNOWLEDGEMENTS

I have spent over two years writing this book. As mentioned elsewhere, I did not make any notes documenting this period of my medical career – I have combined events I remember with some general research. What I recall best are the most unusual, exciting, disappointing, rewarding and surprising.

This has been a learning experience. After writing this book, I have much more respect for the work that is required to actually write a book - from writing the lst page, the lst draft, the many redrafts, the formatting and finally the publishing of the book. I had little appreciation for the process until I went through it myself.

I also have a better sense of what a writer experiences mentally and emotionally. While writing this there were many times that I simply tired of the project and briefly had to set it aside. I now understand why many authors describe writing as a lonely experience. It is – it is just you and your pen and your paper. There is no social interaction. It also requires considerable discipline to continue to completion.

I appreciate now that it takes the contributions of many people to complete a book. It is not a solo endeavour. I have been fortunate to have had the assistance of many individuals.

I would like to thank the following people for their invaluable assistance. If I have omitted anyone's name, I wish to offer my apologies for my oversight.

Firstly, I have to thank Sylvia Jensen and Janet Jeffery for spending many hours typing the various drafts of the manuscript.

ii

I am fortunate to have had the assistance of a group of people I will call "the professionals" – Dr. Leigh Matthews, my editor, who is a member of the English Department at the University College of the Cariboo [to be known as the Thompson Rivers University as of April 2005]; Dwayne Jensen, husband of Sylvia, who is very proficient in computer graphics and who did the formatting; and Christyne Learmonth, my advisor at Trafford Publishing.

Several people have been very generous with their time and read all or parts of the manuscript and provided me with their comments: my wife Lila, Dr. Lyon Appleby, Dr. Ben Dlin, Steve Gittus, and Daryl Parker. Of course any medical or historical errors are my responsibility alone.

The following have been of great assistance during my research and while assembling some of the photographs. They are Gertrude Fraser [former matron at Quesnel General Hospital and wife of Alex Fraser, deceased, former Mayor of Quesnel for several years, and subsequently MLA for the Cariboo in the 1950s and 1960s, including Minister of Highways for several years. The Alex Fraser Bridge in Vancouver is named in his memory], Leslie Middleton, Jean Speare [provided drawing of the Quesnel Clinic and wife of Bill Speare, deceased, former MLA for the Cariboo during the 1950s] and Melanie Hardbattle [St. Paul's Hospital Archives].

Nancy Wise [Sandhill Book Publishing], Ray Foster [Royal Alexandra Hospital]; Joanna Pawlyshyn [Royal Alexandra Hospital]; Marilyn Armstrong [Royal Alexandra Hospital]; Vivian Sinclair [Heritage Publishing Group]; the staff at the Quesnel and District Museum and Archives; the administrative staff at G.R. Baker Memorial Hospital and Bruce Mason [Yale and District Historical Society]; the staff at the College of Physicians and Surgeons of BC library; Zbignien Rabzimowski [Area Manager – Bridges; Lower Mainland District, Ministry of Transportation] and the library staff at Royal Inland Hospital were also very helpful.

My son Phil turned out to be my "boy Friday" – word processing, editing, making suggestions, tracking down information, and introducing me to Dr. Leigh Matthews, and Sylvia and Dwayne Jensen.

I would also like to acknowledge the generosity of the law firm Mair Jensen Blair of Kamloops for allowing my son Phil access to its equipment to photocopy and bind the numerous drafts.

Overall, I can say that although this project proved to be considerably more work than I anticipated, having now completed it I feel that it was well worth the effort. Hopefully, it will give the lay reader some insight into the practice of medicine in the rural areas of BC only 40 to 50 yrs ago. It is amazing the changes that have occurred since then.

As well, this may be of some interest to individuals in the health care profession. Perhaps it may encourage young members of the medical profession to practice in a rural area of this province, at least for part of their career. The recent opening of the school of medicine at the University of Northern BC in Prince George will be a very effective catalyst for this. Lastly, it will help to preserve some of the history of my family.

Len Maher
Feb. 2005
Kamloops, B.C.

PREFACE

I wish to dedicate this book to those men and women who are doing family practice in medicine, surgery and obstetrics in the villages and towns of British Columbia. To me, they are the unsung heroes and heroines of our profession.

I hope my experiences expressed in this book might inspire young graduates to consider seriously spending at least a portion of their professional lives in the rural areas of British Columbia where there is a great need for their expertise.

I would also like to dedicate it to my four children, Phil, Dan, Brenda and Paul.

The initial idea for this book was the brain-child of my eldest son, Phil. If it hadn't been for his continual insistence, I never would have started to write the manuscript. If it hadn't been for his immeasurable help and his persistence, the book never would have been completed.

During the course of a decade in general practice, I saw hundreds of patients in my office, hundreds in the emergency room and labor room of the Quesnel General and G.R. Baker Memorial Hospitals and untold numbers on house calls. Since I kept no diary of these events, I have had to rely on my memory to recount these experiences.

CHAPTER 1: SETTING A GOAL

Why Did I Decide To Study Medicine?

There is not one profession that we need envy: there is none that gives to its students such a good introduction to things as they are.
Earl P. Scarlett M.B.

I have no idea what influenced my decision to study medicine. As I look back, I realize that the odds were not in my favor. No one in my family was a doctor. None of my relatives had gone beyond high school. Both of my parents were printers, having learned their trade after many years of apprenticeship.

I was born at the Royal Alexandra Hospital, in Edmonton, in 1925, two years after the birth of my sister, Eunice. At the time, my family lived in a small bungalow on 110 A Avenue just east of 95th Street. This was one of the districts in Edmonton where the poorer people lived. There were no professional people living there. The majority of the residents were laborers or blue-collar workers.

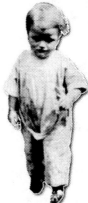

PHOTOGRAGH 1
[Photograph of author at 2 years of age. Taken in 1927 in the backyard of our home in Edmonton, 9267 – 110A Avenue]

Why a boy who was born and raised in this environment should believe that he could become a doctor amazes me when I think of it now. Nevertheless, at the age of ten, when I was asked by anyone what I was going to be when I grew up, I replied that I wanted to be a doctor. As the years went by, I never once changed my mind.

In my early childhood, I had not had any contact with doctors, except for three incidents. My first illness occurred after I had done something foolish. My family was living in Vancouver at the time. We lived in a house in the Kitsilano district on 6th Avenue between Arbutus and Maple Streets. Since our home was seven blocks from Kitsilano Beach, it was a short walk. In those days, there was no fear of young children being abducted by strangers or pedophiles. We felt safe going to and from the beach by ourselves. In the summer time, Eunice and I would walk to the beach practically every day. We would spend the day playing in the sand, running around in the water and playing on the swings and teetertotters in the playground. After playing, exhausted and hungry, we would return home just in time for dinner.

On one sunny day, when I was about 7 years old, I got the brilliant idea that this would be the perfect day to get a suntan. I played in my bathing suit all day and noticed no ill effects until we began our climb up the hill for home. I became aware of a burning sensation on the skin of my shoulders and the backs of my knees. By the time I reached home, the skin was very red and quite uncomfortable. Within a few hours, my shoulders and the backs of my knees were severely blistered. I was experiencing severe pain. This blistering alarmed my grandmother who called a doctor and requested that he come and have a look at me. After examining me, the doctor advised her to keep me in bed, covered with only a cotton sheet, and to apply olive oil to the burned areas several times during the day and night. Fortunately, the burns did not become infected, which could have been serious at that time. The burned areas took about three weeks to heal completely. Needless to say, I have never forgotten that painful episode. To this day, I have a healthy respect for the power of the sun.

My second experience with the medical profession occurred around the age of nine. I had suffered from severe bouts of bronchial asthma. This began shortly after we moved from Edmonton to Vancouver when I was five years old. Prior to this, I had no illnesses. My grandmother had attempted to treat the asthmatic attacks with all of the home remedies known to mankind - oil of eucalyptus on a spoonful of sugar, goose grease applied to the chest, mentholatum in steam, Buckley's Cough Mixture, mustard plasters, cod liver oil, various inhalants and other remedies too numerous to remember. The remedy which I disliked the most was wine of ipecac. The taste of this is difficult to describe, but anyone who has had the pleasure of taking it will never forget it. The purpose of the wine was to act as an emetic, causing the person to vomit in order to clear the throat of excess mucus. It always had the desired effect of causing emesis, but I doubt if it had any effect on the breathing difficulty. I never objected to taking any of these remedies because I knew that my grandmother was doing everything in her power to try to relieve my suffering. Although many of the treatments were unpleasant, none was as bad as the condition being treated.

The only medication which did relieve the dyspnea (difficulty breathing) was adrenalin. A few drops of this was placed into a small atomizer which was used to squirt the medication to the back of the throat and into the trachea. However, only a limited amount of this could be used at intervals due to the effect it had on causing the heart to beat rapidly.

Bronchial asthma is a frightening illness. At the time that I had the problem, it was generally agreed that no one ever died from it. Over the years, it has been shown that this is not true. Statistics in Canada now reveal that several deaths occur from bronchial asthma every year. I spent many a night sitting up in a chair, struggling for air, finally falling asleep from exhaustion.

At the age of ten, I experienced a miracle. My mother took me to see a doctor who was particularly interested in allergic conditions. He carried out skin tests which consisted of making about thirty small incisions on each of my forearms with a scalpel. He then placed a drop of solution containing an allergen onto each incision. There was no reaction at most of the test sites, but there was a marked reaction to the allergen containing cat dander. This indicated a severe sensitivity to cats. We had never owned a cat while living in Edmonton, but had owned one ever since moving to Vancouver. The day following the skin tests, a young man from the SPCA appeared at our home. He played with the family pet for a few minutes, then gently picked him up and placed him into a basket. From that day I have never experienced another attack of asthma. The incidence of asthma in Canada is now at an all-time high. Approximately one person in five is affected. This is mostly due to increased contamination of the air.

Diagnosis and treatment of an allergic problem can be that simple in a small percentage of cases, but more often, it is much more complicated and not so successful. I was one of the fortunate ones. However, I must add that, even now, if I am visiting the home of someone who owns a cat, after a period of about two hours, I will begin to notice itchiness and tearing of my eyes and a slight cough and tightness of my chest. This is the signal for me to leave the house. If I was to remain in that environment, I'm sure I would soon develop severe difficulty in breathing.

My third experience with the medical profession occurred when I was about ten years old. I had had a slight head cold for a couple of days when I began to experience pain in my right ear. Over a period of a few hours, the pain gradually became more severe. It was a continual, throbbing pain deep in the ear canal.

My mother became alarmed at the severity of the pain and decided to phone the family doctor. When he had finished seeing his patients in the office, he drove over to our home to see me. After examining me, he informed my mother that I had a middle ear infection (otitis media) which had reached the stage of abscess formation. He informed her that he would need to make an opening in the eardrum in order to relieve the pressure and allow the pus to drain out of the middle ear. While I lay in bed, the doctor placed a special gauze mask over my nose and mouth. He then poured chloroform from a small brown bottle, drop by drop, until I was soon fast asleep. While I was under the general anaesthetic, he made a small incision (called a myringotomy) through the eardrum with a special tiny, pointed knife. This allowed the pus to drain out of the middle ear and thus relieve the pressure. I was asleep for only a few minutes, but when I awakened, I was completely free of pain.

My mother was then instructed to irrigate my ear canal several times daily. She used a small rubber bulb syringe and a mixture of water and baking soda in order to wash out the canal, thus clearing the canal of pus and debris. After several days, when there was no longer any formation of pus, the irrigations were discontinued. Fortunately, I recovered from this infection with complete healing of the eardrum and no ill effects on my hearing.

Today, this surgical procedure is still carried out fairly frequently. However, when it is performed, it is done by an ear specialist (otologist) with the assistance of a microscope in order to magnify the eardrum adequately so that he is able to do the procedure more precisely. It is also carried out in the operating room of a hospital with an anaesthetist giving the anaesthetic. No doctor today would even consider doing such a procedure at the home of the patient.

Whether these three episodes in my early childhood were instrumental in my decision to become a doctor, I can't really say. I only know that in each case the doctor was able to relieve my suffering. Did this instil in me the desire to be able to relieve the pain and suffering of others?

CHAPTER 2: PRE-MED

Trying To Survive

Medicine is learned at the bedside, not in the classroom.
Sir William Osler

In 1943, at the time that I had completed grade twelve, anyone who wished to carry on into university was required to have his senior matriculation. This meant that he had to write provincial examinations in specific subjects, to pass these examinations and to have at least one hundred credits.

The courses which were required at that time in order to get the one hundred credits were: three years of English, three years of either Latin or French, three years of social studies, two years of physics, two years of chemistry, two years of algebra and one year of geometry and trigonometry. Besides these compulsory courses, we were allowed to take some electives, such as biology, commercial law and bookkeeping. I decided to take three years of Latin instead of French for two reasons: since medical terminology embraces a good deal of Latin, it would be of benefit to me in medical school and since I had not had any French courses in elementary school, I felt that I would be at a disadvantage competing against students who came from French-Canadian families. The choice turned out to be a wise one for me.

I managed not only to pass the provincial examinations, but to achieve an average high enough to allow me to enter the Pre-Medical program at the University of Alberta. This was a two- year program designed specifically for those students who were hoping to carry on into medical school. The required courses in pre-med were: English literature, two years of a foreign language, physics, three chemistry courses, two zoology courses, genetics, statistics and a course in medical Latin and Greek roots.

The course which I enjoyed the most was the one in medical Latin and Greek roots. It was given by Dr. Johns, who was the head of the department of Classics. Dr. Johns had prepared this course himself. It was specifically designed for pre-med students. When Dr. Johns entered the classroom, he would immediately walk up to the blackboard and write a couple of words on the board in Greek. Then he would start his discussion on the terms we would learn for that day. He made the course very interesting and practical.

Non-medical people find medical terms to be both difficult to understand and difficult to pronounce. However, once it is explained in simple language, the confusion disappears. Medical words are composed of Latin and Greek roots which, when combined, define an object quite precisely. For example:

"Gastro" is the Greek word for stomach. "Enteros" is the Greek word for intestine. "Logos" is the Greek word for science. By combining these three words, the word "gastroenterology" is formed, which is the science dealing with diseases of the stomach and intestines. Once a person is acquainted with the basic roots, it is quite simple to understand the meaning of the words and to pronounce them without difficulty.

The most boring and useless course in pre-med was the course in statistics. This course was given by the head of the department of Mathematics. He was an eccentric guy, possibly related to the fact that he was a genius. Most of his first lecture was spent in walking around the perimeter of the class-room while dragging a piece of chalk on the walls. After he had done this a few times, he explained that he had been trying to demonstrate the meaning of infinity. The only thing I can remember learning in this course was that the word "average" really doesn't have any useful function in statistics.

Pre-med was not the most enjoyable period of my life, partly due to the stress of World War II and to uninteresting courses which we were required to take, but mostly due to the fact that it was a weaning-out process for medical school. The stress was intense. The students were under constant pressure not only to pass the courses, but to pass them with high enough marks to be among the select few who would be eligible to continue on into medicine. This never-ending competition was extremely stressful to every student. Some students were so tense as they waited to enter the examination hall that they would jerk if someone accidentally touched them.

During my first year of Pre-Med, when I returned to classes following the Christmas break, I was stunned to find that half of the class was missing. The powers that be had decided that the bottom half of the class would be failed regardless of their marks on the examinations they had written prior to the break. Fortunately, I was somewhere in the top 50% of the class. I can still recall how depressed I felt when I went to the lab in inorganic chemistry and found that my partner and close friend had not made the grade. Those who had failed would automatically go on active service in the armed forces, unless they were considered to be physically or mentally unfit.

In 1944, while in the second year of pre-med, I contracted an infection of the skin of my face. The condition, called impetigo, was caused by the Staphylococcus aureus, a bacterium commonly found on the skin. I spent several days in the students' infirmary at the university. The condition was treated first with a coal-tar ointment, with little improvement. It was then treated with ultraviolet radiation which caused a moderate desquamation (peeling) of the skin accompanied by severe itching. It resembled a bad sunburn.

It took about two weeks for the skin to return to its normal state. Today, this condition could be cleared up with four or five days treatment with penicillin. Although penicillin had been discovered by Fleming in 1928, it was not available for general use in 1944.

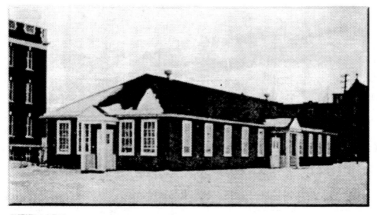

INFIRMARY
A.D. 1943

PHOTO 2 [Infirmary]

During WW II, every able-bodied male university student was obliged to join one of the three branches of the armed forces; army, navy, or air force. I chose to join the University Naval Training Division (UNTD). We were issued regular navy uniforms which had to be worn to classes on Mondays, Wednesdays and Fridays. On these days, after classes, we reported for training sessions, which took place from 6:00 P.M. until 9:00 P.M. During these training periods, we were taught the basics of seamanship.

In the spring, at the completion of the school year, we were taken by train to Vancouver, transferred to the ferry for Victoria, loaded on to covered trucks and taken to the naval barracks at Esquimalt. We slept in hammocks, ate in the regular mess hall and took advanced training at Royal Roads Academy. We did some sailing in the waters off Esquimalt. A few days were spent aboard an old minesweeper travelling from Esquimalt to Powell River and back, allowing us an opportunity to experience life at sea. One night proved to be memorable for those with sensitive semicircular canals (inner ears) when we ran into choppy waters, resulting in some seasickness.

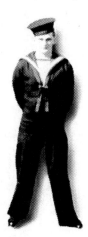

PHOTO 3 [Author in Naval uniform]

All in all, it was an interesting two weeks, which most of us enjoyed. At the completion of the two weeks, we made the return journey to Edmonton where we disbanded for the summer.

Since my family was living in Vancouver at the time, I felt that it did not make sense for me to travel back to Edmonton, purchase a railway ticket and return to Vancouver. I therefore asked to speak to our commanding officer at Esquimalt in order to explain the situation to him. I requested that he allow me to disembark at Vancouver where I lived. He was not very sympathetic. He informed me that since I had left Edmonton with the other trainees that I must return to Edmonton with them. However,

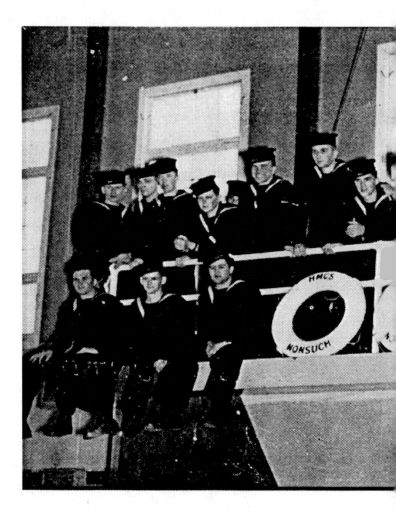

PHOTO 4 [UNTD, author is in front row, 4th from the left]

since I was convinced that this was a foolish thing to do I decided to disobey his orders. When the ferry arrived in Vancouver, instead of marching with the rest of my group from the CPR dock to the CPR rail-

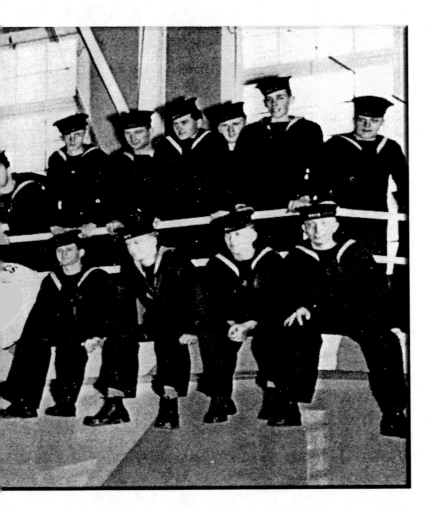

way station, I broke ranks, hailed a taxi and headed for home.

I had just sat down at the kitchen table to enjoy a breakfast of bacon and eggs prepared by my mother when two burly S.P.s (Shore Patrol) appeared at the kitchen door. After verifying that I was seaman Len Maher, they advised me to collect

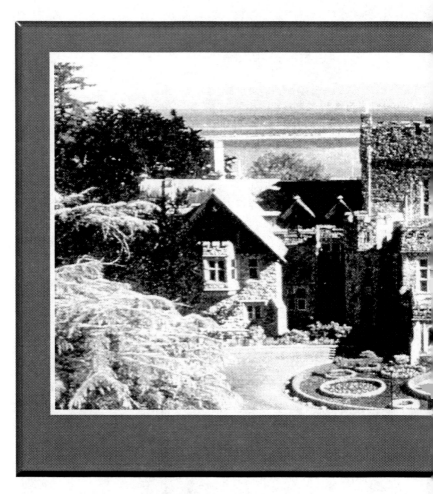

PHOTO 5 [Royal Roads]

my gear and escorted me to the paddy wagon. They drove downtown to naval headquarters, which was located on the ninth floor of the Marine building. The only things missing were the handcuffs and leg irons.

I spoke to the Commanding Officer and explained the reason for my behavior. He informed me that this was a serious matter and that for "jump-

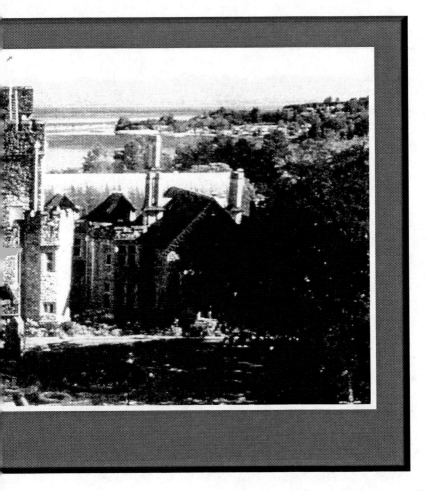

ing ship" and deserting, I could be facing a prison term. After the interview, he left the room and allowed me to sweat for about three hours. During this period I had all sorts of visions as to what my fate would be.

When he finally returned, after what seemed an eternity, he told me that he had decided to overlook my foolish behavior and, with a stern warning, he said that I was free to go home. I decided at that point that I probably wasn't the best of material for

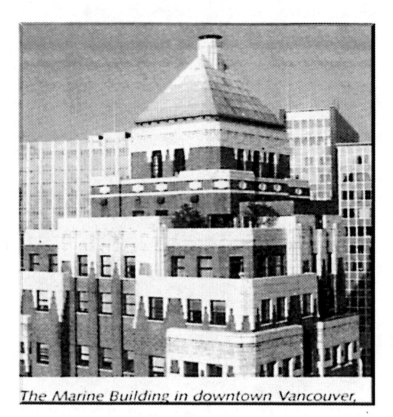
The Marine Building in downtown Vancouver,

PHOTO 6 [Photograph of Marine Building. In l951, this was the tallest building in Vancouver]

the armed forces where orders are to be carried out without asking any questions. I vowed that if I did continue with a career in the navy, I wanted to do so as an officer rather than as an ordinary seaman.

During the war years, although the usual freshman, sophomore, junior and senior proms were held, formal dress was not permitted. There were no tuxedos allowed, women were not permitted to wear full-length formal gowns and corsages were forbidden. This was done in order to show respect for the men and women who were on active service.

During the summer months I was always fortunate in getting a job. This allowed me to earn enough to pay for my tuition, books and part of my room and board. Buying any new clothes was out of the question. On the advice of my mother, my grandfather had bought me a tweed winter coat as a high school graduation present. I wore this coat every winter for the six years while attending university. One of my uncles gave me one of his sports jackets and a pair of shoes when mine began to show signs of wear. I remember being very thankful to receive these gifts.

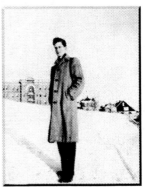

PHOTO 7 [Author dressed in high-school grad present. I wore this coat during the 6 years I attended university]

My first summer's job was at McGavin's Bakery in Vancouver. My job was to grease bread pans. The pans were attached in groups of five and were stacked on pallets to a height of about four feet. A large piece of lard was placed into a small cotton sack. This was held in the right hand, which was scooped through each individual pan. When the fifth pan was greased, all five were flipped off the pile with the left hand. The most important thing was speed. This had to be done as quickly as possible. This was done for eight hours steadily, except for a ten-minute break in the morning and afternoon and a half-hour lunch break. Unfortunately, there was a clock on the wall in the room where I worked. That clock always seemed to be standing still. You can imagine how happy I was when the end of summer finally arrived and I could return to university. There's nothing that can compare to a tough summer job to encourage a person to return to school.

For two summers I worked as a plumber's helper. After the plumber had measured and marked a pipe (galvanized pipes were used in those days), my job was to cut the pipe and then thread the end. I also assisted him in assembling the pipes and with various other jobs, such as assembling four-inch sewage pipes and sealing the joints with oakum and molten lead. This was heavy work at times, but was at least educational.

My experience as a plumber's helper was of benefit to me in the summer of 1945 when I was fortunate to get a job as a pipefitter's helper at the Westcoast Shipyards in Vancouver. The shipyard, located on False Creek, was a very busy place at the time. This is where the famous Victory Ships were being built. The ships were used to transport valuable food, clothing and other supplies from Halifax across the Atlantic to Britain. Many of these ships were sunk by German U-boats with the loss of hundreds of Canadian merchant seamen. It is only recently that these seamen have been given the recognition they deserved.

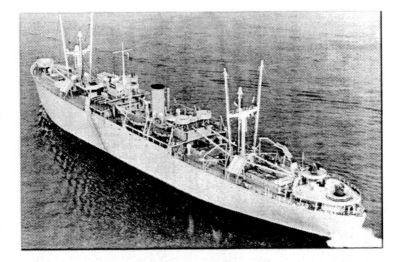

PHOTO 8 [Photograph of a Victory ship]

While I was working at the shipyards, I had the opportunity to observe the shipwrights at their work. I never ceased to be intrigued by the skill of these men. I was especially mesmerized by their manual dexterity in using marlin spikes to join cables, make knots and eyelets. It was obvious to me that these men had acquired these skills through many years of training and hard work. I was paid 75¢ an hour for my work in the shipyards. I felt that this was a terrific wage at that time.

At the time that I worked as a plumber's helper, galvanized pipes were being used for hot and cold water. I learned how to measure these pipes accurately, and how to cut, ream and thread them. I also became quite skilful at using pipe wrenches.

Years later, when galvanized pipes were replaced with copper, it was not difficult to teach myself how to work with these using a blow torch and solder. When copper piping was replaced with plastic, plumbing became even easier.

During the summer of 1946, I got a job as a painter's helper painting the outside of houses, apartments and commercial buildings in Vancouver. One of the buildings we had to paint was Carling's Brewery situated on 12th Avenue near Connaught Park.

We had a fifteen-minute break in the morning and afternoon. The other painters would have a free glass of beer during these breaks, but since I did not drink, I would usually wander around and watch the workmen in the brewery. One day I stopped to watch a man whose job was to take the used, empty bottles out of boxes and place them on a conveyor belt. The belt would carry them along to a machine which washed them. I began talking to this man and learned that he had been doing this job for "twenty years". I found it hard to believe. Unless a person has actually had a job where he has to keep up with moving machinery he has no idea how monotonous and tedious this type of work can be. I had witnessed this same sort of thing the year I had worked in the bakery where men had to keep up to a machine while they handled the rolls of dough that would eventually become loaves of bread. Apparently, many of these people prefer to have a job where they do not have to think, have very little responsibility and do not have to give the job a thought once they stop work at five o'clock. After seeing and speaking to this man, I was more resolved than ever to continue on at university.

In the summers of 1947 and 1948, I helped to paint the outside of the houses in Powell River. At that time, Powell River was a company town so all of the houses were owned by the Powell River Paper Company. Besides painting the houses, we painted the inside of a second paper mill which had just been completed. When the second mill went into production, producing newsprint, the company became the largest paper mill in the British Empire.

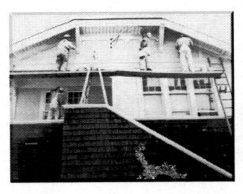

PHOTO   9 [Painters, Powell River]

The heat to which we were subjected while painting the ceiling of this building (while the machinery was running) could be endured for only a few minutes at a time before requiring a break. The fumes of sulphur trioxide in the air in the vicinity of the mill were so bad that a person's lungs felt raw from inhaling them.

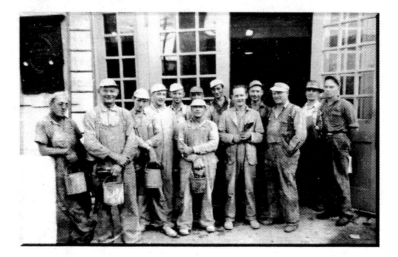

PHOTO 10 [Painting crew, Powell River; author is missing]

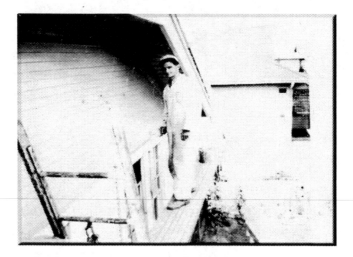

PHOTO   11 [Author painting house in Powell River]

At the time that I was painting, oil-based paints were being used exclusively. Rollers had not been invented. We used 3-inch brushes to paint ceilings and walls and 1 1/2inch brushes to paint the trim around windows. We used 4 inch brushes to paint the outside of houses.

Years later, when rollers were invented for painting large, flat surfaces and water-based paints became available, painting became considerably easier.

I was taught the basics of how to hold a paintbrush properly (you would be surprised how many people do not know this basic principle). I was shown how to use a paint pot to paint from, rather than the can in which paint is purchased (most people paint right out of the can purchased from the painting store). I learned how to cut along an edge accurately and skillfully.

I was also instructed in how to use an extension ladder safely, and how to use ladder jacks and swing stages. Many of the skills taught to me by the men I worked with were used many times over the years while painting my own home.

Since all of my summer jobs involved quite a bit of physical exertion, I was always in pretty good physical condition. However, I was always happy to see the end of summer so that I could get back to school. By the same token, when spring arrived and our final exams were over, I was mentally exhausted and happy to have a break from the intensity of study.

During the six years that I attended university, I did not have what could be called a vacation. I went from university to work and back to university. However, there is an old saying that "change is as good as a rest" and it seemed to work for me – not that I had any choice. During the six years that I attended university, I was not able to get home to Vancouver during a single Christmas break. The cost of the train fare was simply too much for my budget. Most of the time I walked two or three miles back and forth to university in order to save on streetcar fare. It was good exercise and, by the time I arrived at classes or clinics, I was wide awake, especially in the winter months. Walking over the High-Level Bridge on a cold, windy, winter day was enough to awaken anyone.

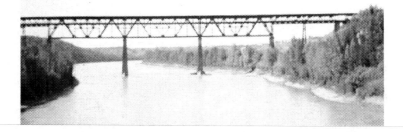

PHOTO 12 [High Level Bridge]

Although I was fortunate to be able to attend university during the war years, it was not easy. The fear of failing was forever present. There was always a sense of guilt whenever I took time off from my studies in order to relax or participate in some activity which was non-academic. However, I usually took off parts of Saturdays and Sundays to pursue extra-curricular activities.

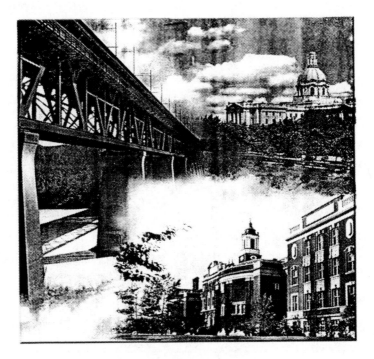

PHOTO 13 [Photo showing high-level bridge, Legislative building, Medical Building]

CHAPTER 3: MEDICAL SCHOOL

The Real Studying Begins

The practice of medicine is an art based on science.
Sir William Osler

I considered pre-med to be a stepping stone to my real purpose in life, a necessary hurtle which had to be endured. After thousands of hours of study, dozens of nights of sleep deprivation and doing without many of the pleasures enjoyed by my non-university friends, I entered the first year of medical school along with thirty-five other students. Receiving my letter of acceptance in 1945 was one of the most exciting moments of my life.

Something which became apparent from the first day of medical school was the difference in attitude of the professors in the faculty of medicine towards the students. It was obvious that they wanted us to succeed and did everything they could to help us. We were no longer undergoing a weeding-out process. The message was clear that we had faced the challenge and had proven ourselves capable of the task.

Although the volume and complexity of the work was considerably greater than it had been in pre-med, this was offset by the fact that the work was more interesting, practical and goal-oriented. There was a light beginning to appear at the end of the tunnel, although it was still a long way off.

The first two years of medical school were devoted to the basic sciences. The basic sciences consisted of gross anatomy, microscopic anatomy (histology), developmental anatomy (embryology), neuroanatomy, physiology, biochemistry, bacteriology (microbiology) and pharmacology.

Every one of these courses was tough, consisted of lectures and labs, and was loaded with material which had to be mastered. Medical school is no place for the person who is not able to commit thousands of facts to memory. The modern concept that students do not need to memorize anything will shock anyone entering medical school. The ability to memorize is an absolute essential in achieving a medical degree.

Our academic year always began the day after the Labour Day holiday and ended on the last day of May, following final examinations. The exams consisted of three-hour written exams and two hour lab exams. We were always the first students to return to university in the fall and the last to leave in the spring.

From Monday until Friday, our day started at 8:00 A.M. and went to Noon. We had one hour for lunch and then went from 1:00 P.M. to 5:00 P.M. with lectures or labs. On Saturdays, we had classes from 8:00 A.M. until Noon. At the completion of the day, we went home for dinner and then studied for the remainder of the evening.

There were thirty-six members in my first-year medical class. The majority of these students had come through the pre-med program. Four of them were women: Maimie Bailey, Margery Fraser, Margaret Hunter and Sheila Sheehan. Eight members of the class had completed science degrees prior to the war, had joined the armed forces and were now returning to university to complete their studies. These were the older and more mature members of the class.

On Saturday evenings, my girlfriend (and future wife) Connie Eccles and I would either go ice-skating at the outdoor rink on 112th Street and Jasper Avenue, go to a movie or go dancing at the Barn, a dance hall downtown where we could dance all evening for one dollar.

We also managed to go to a couple of the major dances at the university and to the dinner and dance which was held on "Color Night". Color Night was the special event held near the end of the school year when the athletes, male and female, were given special recognition. Besides playing some medical-school hockey, I was quite active in the boxing club. I won the intercollegiate boxing championships in the years 1944, 1945 and 1946, for which I received a 6-inch letter the first year and bars to go with it in subsequent years. In 1946, I was awarded the Beaumont Trophy for the best record in boxing, and also the Wynichuk Trophy for having done the most for the boxing club. Color Night was a big night for me in 1946.

Pat Johnston would have been proud of me if he had been living at the time. Pat and I had gone

The boxing season was brought to a close with the Assault-at-Arms against the University of Saskatchewan.

Ray Fleming won his bout when Saskatchewan failed to produce an exponent of the fistic art in the heavyweight division. Rough light-heavy Eldor Berg flashed a beautiful right hook to put Bob Gray from U. of S. away in the third on a T.K.O. In the middleweight set-to Jack Perry, club coach, took a crowd-pleasing but unscientific bout after cutting up his opponent severely, winning a unanimous decision.

Laurie MacLean outpointed Johnny Galon of Saskatchewan in the welterweight division on a split decision. Feature of this go was the collapse of the ring during one of MacLean's more ambitious attacks upon Galon. Novice Bill Parsons of Alberta fought a very game but losing battle against smooth Horace Beach, voted best boxer of the night, to go out by the TKO route in the fourth round. The featherweight title went to Alberta on a unanimous decision as fast, talented Lennie Maher bested Frank Howarth of Saskatchewan.

Our Club claimed the Howe trophy by defeating five of the six Saskatchewan boxers. The Beaumont trophy was awarded to Eldor Berg for the fine sportsmanship and boxing ability that he has shown throughout the boxing season.

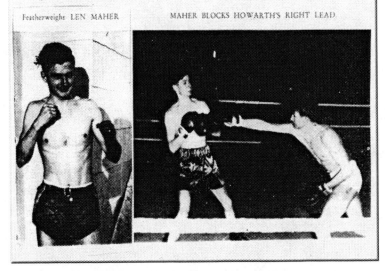

Featherweight LEN MAHER   MAHER BLOCKS HOWARTH'S RIGHT LEAD

PHOTO 14 [Boxing tournament against the University of Saskatchewan]

through elementary and high schools together and were very close friends. He had won the boxing championship for the province of Alberta when he was in his early teens.

When I was about thirteen, I asked Pat if he would teach me to box. He said he'd be happy to

31

teach me what he could. At that time Pat had a job helping an auctioneer on Saturdays. He managed to get me hired as his assistant. The auctions took place in a large warehouse that was located on Jasper Avenue just west of 95th street. When the auctions were over for the day, we would go up to the second floor of the building where there was plenty of open space. He taught me the proper stance, how to hold my hands and arms, how to move about the ring, how to throw the different punches and many other things. He was a great instructor and taught me everything I know about boxing. While I was in high school, I managed to win the championship for the city of Edmonton.

When Pat had completed grade eleven at St. Joseph's High School, he decided to join the Army rather than continue into grade twelve. It wasn't long before he was a paratrooper and was shipped overseas. Several months later I received a phone call from his oldest sister Pauline informing me that Pat had been killed in action while participating in a raid over France. It was a great shock to me. He was the first of a number of friends I would lose in the war.

We are forever hearing of women being discriminated against at the universities and in the various professions. I was not aware of this happening when I was in medical school. At a recent class reunion, I asked Dr. Margaret Hunter, a member of the class and a retired pediatrician, if she had felt any discrimination when she was going through medical school.

Her reply was an emphatic "*NO*". "*As a matter of fact*", she said, "*we always felt very protected by the male members of the class. We were always treated fairly and with the same respect as*

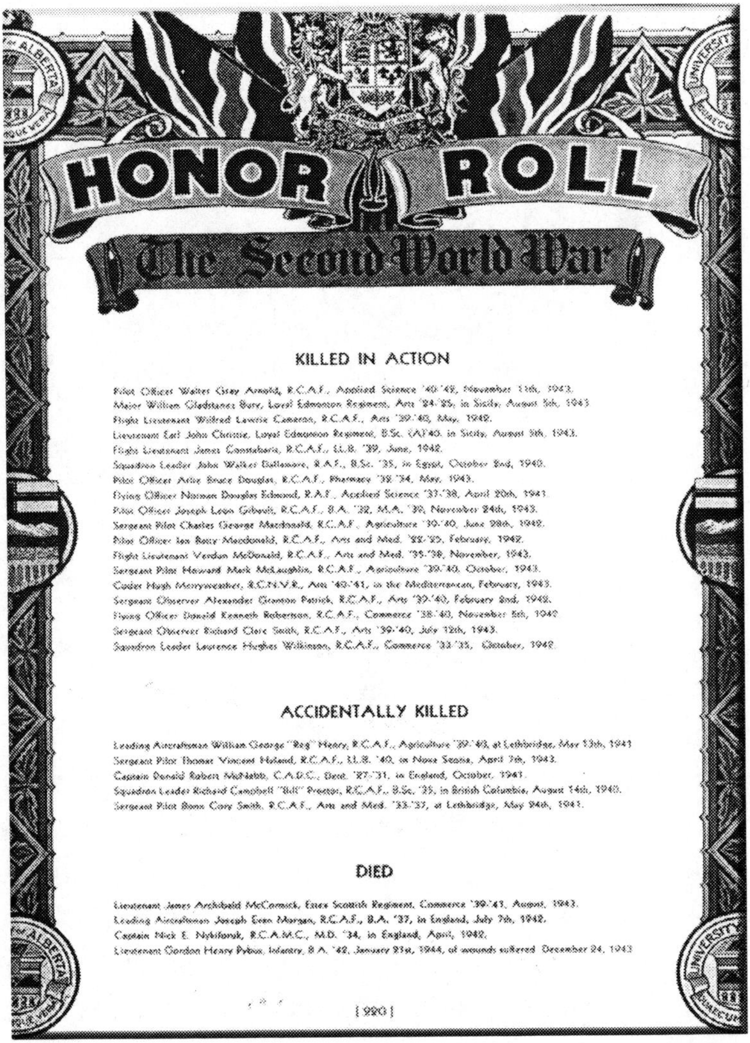

HONOR ROLL

The Second World War

KILLED IN ACTION

Pilot Officer Walter Gray Arnold, R.C.A.F., Applied Science '40-'42, November 13th, 1943.
Major William Gladstanes Bury, Loyal Edmonton Regiment, Arts '24-'25, in Sicily, August 5th, 1943.
Flight Lieutenant Wilfred Lowrie Cameron, R.C.A.F., Arts '39-'40, May, 1942.
Lieutenant Earl John Christie, Loyal Edmonton Regiment, B.Sc. (A)'40, in Sicily, August 5th, 1943.
Flight Lieutenant James Constabaris, R.C.A.F., LL.B. '39, June, 1942.
Squadron Leader John Walker Dallamore, R.A.F., B.Sc. '35, in Egypt, October 2nd, 1940.
Pilot Officer Arlie Bruce Douglas, R.C.A.F., Pharmacy '33-'34, May, 1943.
Flying Officer Norman Douglas Edmond, R.A.F., Applied Science '37-'38, April 20th, 1941.
Pilot Officer Joseph Leon Gibault, R.C.A.F., B.A. '32, M.A. '39, November 24th, 1943.
Sergeant Pilot Charles George Macdonald, R.C.A.F., Agriculture '39-'40, June 28th, 1942.
Pilot Officer Ian Ross Macdonald, R.C.A.F., Arts and Med. '33-'35, February, 1942.
Flight Lieutenant Verdun McDonald, R.C.A.F., Arts and Med. '35-'38, November, 1943.
Sergeant Pilot Howard Mark McLaughlin, R.C.A.F., Agriculture '39-'40, October, 1943.
Cadet Hugh Merryweather, R.C.N.V.R., Arts '40-'41, in the Mediterranean, February, 1943.
Sergeant Observer Alexander Gowan Patrick, R.C.A.F., Arts '39-'40, February 2nd, 1942.
Flying Officer Donald Kenneth Robertson, R.C.A.F., Commerce '38-'40, November 5th, 1942.
Sergeant Observer Richard Clore Smith, R.C.A.F., Arts '39-'40, July 12th, 1943.
Squadron Leader Laurence Hughes Wilkinson, R.C.A.F., Commerce '33-'35, October, 1942.

ACCIDENTALLY KILLED

Leading Aircraftman William George "Reg" Henry, R.C.A.F., Agriculture '39-'40, at Lethbridge, May 13th, 1941.
Sergeant Pilot Thomas Vincent Holand, R.C.A.F., LL.B. '40, in Nova Scotia, April 7th, 1943.
Captain Donald Robert McNabb, C.A.D.C., Dent. '27-'31, in England, October, 1941.
Squadron Leader Richard Campbell "Bill" Proctor, R.C.A.F., B.Sc. '35, in British Columbia, August 14th, 1940.
Sergeant Pilot Ross Cory Smith, R.C.A.F., Arts and Med. '33-'37, at Lethbridge, May 24th, 1941.

DIED

Lieutenant James Archibald McCormick, Essex Scottish Regiment, Commerce '39-'43, August, 1943.
Leading Aircraftman Joseph Evan Morgan, R.C.A.F., B.A. '37, in England, July 7th, 1942.
Captain Nick E. Nybiforuk, R.C.A.M.C., M.D. '34, in England, April, 1942.
Lieutenant Gordon Henry Pybus, Infantry, B.A. '42, January 23rd, 1944, of wounds suffered December 24, 1943.

[220]

PHOTO 15 [Honor Roll list taken from the 1945 University of Alberta Yearbook listing War casualties]

any other member". I can't say how pleased I was to hear this. However, I learned recently that there was a quota on the number of female students who were allowed to enter the first year of medicine. In our year, it apparently was four.

The first two years of medical school were devoted to the study of the basic sciences. If there is one year of medical school which stands out from all of the others, for me, it is the first year. There was a feeling of excitement and adventure.

The centre of our lives for the first two years was the medical building, a large, impressive structure situated near the centre of the campus. We had to climb several steps to reach the front door of the building. After passing through this door, up a few more steps, across a hallway, then passing through another door, we entered the sanctum sanctorum of the medical building, the Conn Room. This room had been dedicated to the memory of Dr. Conn, a deceased professor of Obstetrics and Gynecology. Only medical students were allowed into this room. It was a large room with a carpeted floor and a huge fireplace at one end. It contained quite a few comfortable chairs. There was a small room off the main one containing a desk and telephone. Between classes, and at lunch time, students from every year would congregate in this room to relax, make phone calls, shoot the breeze and even play a bit of poker. It was in this room that we were able to meet many of the students who were in the second, third or fourth years of the program.

There was always a cheery atmosphere in the Conn Room. Advice from senior students was often sought and freely given. Over a short period of a few weeks, a strong feeling of camaraderie developed among all of the students.

The first morning of medical school will always remain memorable for me. Dr. Rawlinson, who taught the course in gross anatomy, gave his first lecture. He described the general layout of the anatomy room, how the cadavers had been willed to the university by the deceased or their relatives and how fortunate we were to have the privilege of being able to study anatomy by personal dissection. We were advised to show the utmost respect for the cadavers. Frivolity would not be tolerated. He then described in detail the dissection we would be carrying out that morning. We were divided into groups of four and taken to the dissecting room.

The first thing to strike our senses was the strong odour of formaldehyde which had been injected into the cadavers as a preservative. Four students were assigned to each table, one pair on each side. My partner was Jim Wesolowski, one of the two students in my high-school class who had continued on to university. We were on the right side of the table. The couple occupying the left side of the table were Ben Dlin and Eli Schecter. We learned that our cadaver had been a patient at the Oliver Mental Hospital for many years and that his relatives had been willing to donate his body to the medical school in order to help in the education of the students. In keeping with a custom that had been passed down through the ages, we agreed to christen our cadaver "Floyd".

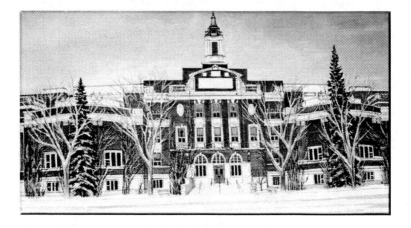

PHOTO 16 [Photo of Medical School Building at the University of Alberta as it was when the author attended school]

The dissection of the first day started with the chest wall, the skin, sub-cutaneous nerves and muscles. From there we continued into the axilla (armpit) in order to identify the main bundle of nerves which supply the upper extremity (the brachial plexus). We studied the muscles, their origins and insertions, the tendons, ligaments, nerves and blood vessels of the upper arm, forearm and hand.

On completion of the dissection of the upper extremity, we turned to the lower extremity, which we studied in similar detail. We then turned our attention to the abdomen. The muscles of the abdominal wall were dissected, the peritoneal cavity was opened, and systematic dissection of the organs, such as the stomach, small and large intestines, liver, spleen, pancreas, kidneys, ureters, adrenal glands, the major arteries, veins, and nerves, were carried out.

From the abdominal cavity, it was a short route to the pelvis, which contains the uterus, ovaries, uterine tubes and vagina in the female, the prostate, penis and related structures in the male, and the anal canal and anus in both sexes.

After completing the dissection of the pelvis, we then moved on to the thorax (chest). The intricate anatomy of the rib cage was studied. After opening the chest, we dissected the diaphragm, heart, lungs, bronchi, esophagus, plus the major arteries, veins and nerves. The final and most difficult part of the dissection was reserved for the last, the head and neck. The muscles, nerves and arteries of the face were identified along with the parotid and submaxillary salivary glands. The external nose and nasal cavity, the eyeballs and muscles controlling their movement, and the external, middle and inner ears were studied. The thyroid gland with the adjacent muscles, arteries, veins and nerves were carefully dissected.

We were required to learn in great detail all of the parts of the skeleton, which included the skull, the vertebrae, ribs, pelvic bones and bones of the arms and legs, plus all of their associated joints.

Ben and Eli were two of the four members of my class who were Jewish. The others were Bob

Paradny and Juda Busheiken. Juda was a very good student who came from Calgary. In the early part of the first year, he unfortunately developed a condition known as "malignant hypertension", to which he succumbed.

Malignant hypertension is a condition in which the patient develops an alarming elevation of his blood pressure. This is accompanied by severe headaches, vomiting, visual disturbances, transient blindness and paralyses. The condition progresses to convulsions, stupor and coma. At that time, there was no specific treatment available for this condition, so the interval from onset until death was a short one.

I was not aware of this at the time, nor for many years after graduation, but apparently there was a quota on the number of Jews who were to be admitted into the first year of medicine. In our year, it turned out to be four. If I had known of this at the time, I would have been upset because I am against any type of a quota system. I believe that students should be chosen purely on the basis of their ability. Sex, language, colour, and so on, should not enter the picture. At the present time in Canada, there are quota systems which apply to some medical schools and law schools, the R.C.M.P. and the Armed Forces. Natives, Francophones and females are given preference over some other students who might be equally or more qualified.

Today, in many areas of endeavour, the person discriminated against the most appears to be the white, anglo-saxon male. This represents reverse discrimination in my opinion and is wrong. I am surprised that it has not been challenged as contrary to the Charter of Rights and Freedoms.

More hours were devoted to the study of gross anatomy than to any other subject. Dissection began every morning at 8:00 A.M. and continued until 12 Noon. The course was a full year course. At the completion of each morning in the lab, we scrubbed our hands with soap and water. In contrast to medical students today who use surgical gloves to do their dissections, we used our bare hands. In spite of the hard scrubbing, it was not possible to remove the odor of formaldehyde which was quite noticeable while we were eating our sandwiches at lunchtime. It took time to get used to this. Despite that smell, I consider myself fortunate to have been able to study anatomy in such minute detail. Much of the knowledge remains with me today, over fifty years later.

I used to wonder how the bones of the skeleton were treated in such a manner that they became absolutely clean of any soft tissue, smooth and white. One day this question was answered for me when I happened to glance into a small room which was located just off the main dissecting room. As I looked into the room, I observed a large wooden box in the centre of the room. The box contained a whole skeleton, the remains of a course dissection. As I looked closer, I found that there were dozens of maggots at work cleaning the soft tissue from the bones. This feast continued until every bone was stripped of any vestige of muscle, tendon, fat or any other soft tissue. It was an awesome sight to observe.

Today, students spend relatively less time on anatomy, mainly because the amount of material to be covered in other courses has become so vast that it would be impossible to dedicate so much time to one subject. At the present time, medical students are not required to learn the minute detail in anatomy that we did. In some schools, dissection is actually carried out by a prosector such as a post-graduate student, a resident in surgery or one of the professors. The dissected parts are then demonstrated to the students who are gathered in small groups. I feel sorry for these students because the dissecting lab was one of the main features of medical school which gave the student the feeling of being "almost a doctor". It was, without a doubt, one of the highlights of being a medical student.

In the first year of medical school, we lost three members of our class. Although they were good students and had worked hard, they were not able to keep up with the volume of work which had to be learned. When I returned to university in the fall to start the second year, I was saddened to learn that they were no longer with us.

In medical school, there was no way a student could fail a subject and repeat it. There was no such thing as supplemental exams nor summer school courses. The only way for the student to continue was to be allowed to repeat the whole year. This did happen occasionally. One of the members of my class did poorly in the third year. He had joined our first-year class in 1945 after having been in the air force. He had been a tail-gunner and had completed over thirty missions. It was rare for a tail-gunner to last that long. They were usually shot down long before that. He was quite nervous due to the extremely stressful experience as a tail-gunner. In spite of hard work on his part, he was unable to absorb all of the material required in the third year. This year was an overwhelming year as far as the volume of work was concerned. He was allowed to repeat the third year, which he did successfully. I have to hand him a lot of credit. He had a wife and three children at the time which made it much more difficult for him. He finished the fourth year, interned for one year and became a very good general practitioner in a small town in Eastern Alberta.

CHAPTER 4: MORE BASIC SCIENCES

Work, Work and More Work

More things are missed by not looking than by not knowing.

Sir William Osler

Although gross anatomy was the major basic science to which we devoted a good deal of our time in the first year, there were several other basic sciences which had to be learned over a two-year period. The understanding of these subjects was essential in order to appreciate the clinical courses which we would be taught in the third and fourth years.

Microscopic anatomy, or histology, is the science which deals with those parts of anatomy which are beyond the reach of the naked eye. Dr. Shaner, the head of the department of anatomy, taught this course. He had prepared a series of slides of the various tissues of the body. Each student was given a box of about one hundred slides, along with a microscope which was for his personal use for an entire year. We studied these slides, going over them repeatedly, until we knew the characteristics of each and every tissue and organ in the body.

We studied epithelial cells, which formed the skin and mucous membranes, cells which formed the various glands found in the body, blood cells and the cells of bone, fat, muscle and cartilage. We became familiar with structures such as nerve cells and nerve fibers, blood vessels, the heart and other organs and various glands of the body. We would test each other by putting slides under our microscopes, and asking a fellow student to describe what he saw in detail. It wasn't long before we could describe every slide without hesitation.

Developmental anatomy, or embryology, is the science which deals with the development of the human being from the time of fertilization of the ovum by the spermatozoon to the time of complete development of the infant. As well as giving us lectures on the subject, Dr. Shaner had prepared a series of slides which depicted the embryo in its various stages of development.

Besides explaining the normal development of the fetus, embryology provides explanations for abnormalities which occur when the normal process goes awry. It gives us a reason for such conditions as hare lip and cleft palate, hydrocephalus, spina bifida, congenital heart disease in its various forms, Siamese twins and many other conditions. A sound knowledge of embryology is essential to training in all branches of medicine, but especially in anatomy, surgery and pathology.

Neuro-anatomy refers to the study of the structure of the nervous system. This is the most highly organized system in the body. The essential anatomy of the brain and spinal cord was studied microscopically by means of cross-sections which had been specially prepared, stained and transferred to slides. Detailed knowledge of this anatomy is essential in order to appreciate the signs and symptoms of the various injuries and diseases of the nervous system. The specialties of neurology and neurosurgery represent excellent examples of applied anatomy and physiology of the nervous system. Neuro-anatomy was a separate half-year course which we took in the second year of medical school. It was a very difficult course.

Physiology is the science which deals with the "functions" of the various parts and organs of the body. We studied the various systems of the body in great detail. The labs consisted mostly in the study of the effect of various drugs on the heart of the frog. For our experiments, we used large frogs which were pinned to flat boards by passing straight pins through their four legs. The chest was then opened with pointed scissors in order to expose the heart. A small hook was passed through the tip of the heart and then connected to a system of levers. This would allow us to register the heartbeat on a rotating drum. By applying various drugs directly to the heart, we could determine the effect of the drugs on the heart. When the experiments for the day were completed, we would kill the frog by passing a long needle down the spinal canal of the frog, a process known as "pithing". This destroyed the brain and spinal cord.

Bacteriology is the science which deals with the study of bacteria. Bacteria are one-celled organisms that are too small to be seen with the naked eye. The bacteria which we studied were those which cause various diseases in man. They live and grow in the blood, bones and soft tissues and may produce poisonous waste products known as toxins.

In order to study bacteria, it is necessary to grow them on certain food substances prepared in the laboratory. These special foods are called culture media. The bacteria to be studied are smeared on to glass slides, allowed to dry, then stained with special stains. By studying these slides under the microscope, it is possible to determine the type of bacterium which is present. There are dozens of bacteria which cause various diseases or infections such as: boils, abscesses, tuberculosis, diphtheria, tetanus, typhoid fever, gonorrhea, meningitis, pneumonia, leprosy, plague and many others.

Our bacteriology course was lab-oriented. We studied the methods of growing bacteria on special cultures, transferring them to slides, staining them with special stains and finally identifying them under the microscope. We had dozens of slides and were expected to be able to identify the various bacteria on these slides and the infections or diseases which they caused. The course was a very practical and interesting one.

Biochemistry is the science which deals with chemical processes that take place in the human body. In this course we studied such things as carbohydrates, proteins, fats, vitamins, minerals, enzymes and hormones. Although we did not take a specific course in nutrition, we studied many aspects of this in our courses in biochemistry and physiology.

In one of our labs we were demonstrating how urine can be checked for the presence of sugar. Sugar should not be present in normal urine. After we had completed the test and demonstrated various amounts of sugar in the different specimens of urine, the lab instructor remarked to the class that there was a far simpler and quicker way of testing for sugar. Having said that, he dipped a finger into a specimen of urine, then put the finger in his mouth. Of course we were all shocked when we saw him do this. As we stood there in amazement, he remarked "*of course you didn't notice that I put my index finger into the specimen of urine, but placed my middle finger into my mouth*". On another occasion, our experiment for the day was to test the gastric juice present in the stomach. In order to do this each of us had to obtain a sample of the fluid from our own stomachs. This necessitated our passing a large gastric tube into the stomach by putting the end of the tube into our mouths, pushing it to the back of the throat and then gradually feeding it down the esophagus until it entered the stomach. This sounds like a pretty simple procedure, but for those with a strong gag reflex, it can be a formidable task. Some of the students were able to do it without batting an eye. For others, numerous attempts were required before they were able to swallow the tube amidst violent gagging. There was one member of the class who, try as he might, was unable to swallow the tube. His gag reflex was so strong that he could get the tube only so far before he would throw up. He finally had to give up in defeat.

We were given a special lab course in parasitology by Dr. Shaw, head of the department of bacteriology. A parasite is a plant or animal which lives upon another living organism. In this course, we studied many parasites which cause diseases in humans. Most of these diseases occurred only in tropical countries and included conditions such as malaria, sleeping sickness, amebiasis, leishmaniasis, toxoplasmosis, giardiasis and trichomoniasis. We studied these organisms under the microscope, giving us a better appreciation of the disease process.

Malaria is a good example of a parasitic disease. It is transmitted to humans by the bite of the anopheles mosquito. When an infected mosquito bites a person, it injects a large number of parasites into the blood stream. Each parasite attaches itself to a red blood cell. The various stages of growth of the parasite within the blood cell can be seen by taking a sample of blood, placing it on a glass slide and staining it with a special stain. We studied special slides showing the various stages of the parasite. Malaria remains the major infectious disease problem in the world.

During this course, we also studied diseases caused by various worms, such as hookworm, tapeworm, round worms and pin worm. The pin worm is a very common intestinal parasite, especially in children. When passed in the stool, it resembles a motile piece of white thread. When the worms are passed out of the anus, they cause intense itching. The diagnosis is made by making a smear from the anal region and examining it for the eggs. The study of various worms which infest man is a fascinating study.

Pharmacology is the science which deals with the study of drugs. Since a drug is broadly defined as any chemical agent that affects living processes, the subject of pharmacology is obviously quite extensive. However, the physician is interested primarily in drugs that are useful in the prevention, diagnosis and treatment of human disease. The course dealt with the history of drugs, the sources, physical and chemical properties and the biochemical and physiological effects. When studying drugs, it is important to know the methods of absorption, distribution in the body, main site of action, route of excretion, the optimum dosage and toxic effects. Relatively few drugs used today are still obtained from natural sources and most of these are highly purified or standardized and differ very little from synthetic chemicals. We were fortunate in that our instructor had a medical degree and had had some experience in general practice. He also had a degree in pharmacology, which made him very knowledgeable in the subject. Therefore, he was able to make the course both interesting and practical.

The study of drugs is such a vast subject that it is essential to have the material well organized. Drugs were divided into major groups according to the systems and organs they acted upon, such as: the central nervous system, the cardiovascular system, blood vessels, the respiratory system, the kidneys, and the blood cells. They were also divided into groups according to specific functions, such as: antihistamines, anaesthetic agents, chemotherapeutic agents, hormones and vitamins. When it came to studying individual drugs, a routine was usually followed, which included: the history of the drug, its source, preparations, routes of administration (oral, inhalation, absorption through the skin or mucous membranes), injection (subcutaneous, intramuscular, intravenous), distribution of the drug through the body, action on cells, tissues, organs, method of excretion, therapeutic dosage, possible interactions with other drugs, complications and toxic reactions. When I studied pharmacology in the 1940s, it seemed to be quite a difficult course. Today, with new drugs appearing almost daily, it must be a tough subject for medical students.

CHAPTER 5: THE CLINICAL YEARS

Beginning to Feel Like Real Doctors

Listen to the patient. He is telling you what the problem is.

Sir William Osler

Although I mentioned earlier that the first two years of medical school were devoted entirely to the basic sciences, that wasn't completely true. During the second half of the second year, we were given a course in physical diagnosis by Dr. Ken Hamilton, a cardiologist and former Rhodes Scholar. The course was an interesting introduction to clinical medicine. The first thing we covered was the art of taking a history from the patient. This still remains the most important first step when seeing a patient for a medical or surgical problem. We were instructed to let the patient tell his story, in his own words, as to why he came to see the doctor. We were cautioned not to coach the patient nor to attempt to put words into his mouth. When the patient had finished telling his story, only then were we to begin asking him questions directly related to his complaints. From here we proceeded to inquire about his past illnesses, accidents and surgical procedures. History of family illnesses was then discussed. It was important to ask about any medications that he might be taking at that time. We finished by asking him specific questions relating to the various systems of the body. Only when the history was completed, did we begin with our examination, which was carried out in a systematic manner in order to avoid missing anything of significance.

William Osler, the most famous of all Canadian physicians, made the following statement during one of his bedside teaching sessions: *"More things are missed by not looking than by not knowing"*. He was stressing the importance of carefully observing the patient. Of course, if a doctor does not know what to look for, he could easily miss an important sign even if it was staring him in the face.

The concept of looking at the whole patient and not just one small area (Holistic medicine) is not new, although there seems to be many people today who think they have coined a new phrase and a new method of practising medicine. Holistic medicine has been practiced by the medical profession for centuries.

During our sessions with Dr. Hamilton, we saw many patients with various diseases in order to demonstrate the signs which accompany these diseases. Only by seeing patients with signs and having them demonstrated by a knowledgeable instructor can the student come to appreciate their significance. In order to acquire a good medical education, it is necessary to see thousands of patients with a variety of medical and surgical conditions. This knowledge cannot be adequately obtained from a text book.

It is ironic that Dr. Hamilton, a heart specialist, developed coronary artery disease. (The coronary arteries are the arteries which nourish the heart muscle.) As a result of this, he developed heart block (a very slow heart rate caused by disease of the conduction system of the heart). Heart block was the cause of his death, a condition which, today, would have been easily treated with a pacemaker.

The third and fourth years of medical school were called the clinical years. This was the time that we really began to see patients.

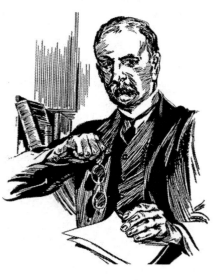

PHOTO 17 [Photo of Sir William Osler]

In order to do this, it was necessary for us to have proper tools. We were required to purchase a stethoscope and a diagnostic set. The diagnostic set contained an otoscope to examine the ears of patients and an ophthalmoscope to examine the retinae of the eyes. We also needed a percussion hammer to test for reflexes. We carried the stethoscope in one of the pockets of our jacket but were usually careful to make sure that a little bit of it could be seen. This was the sign that we were senior medical students. There is no doubt that there was considerable pride in being a medical student.

The mornings of the third and fourth years of medical school were spent at one of the four teaching hospitals in the city. Each morning we saw patients who had been specifically selected to demonstrate the symptoms and signs of a particular disease. These were pointed out to us by the clinical instructor or professor. Our class was divided into groups with six students to a group. My group consisted of McCoy, McLean, McCauley, McCracken, Nattress and Maher. The group would meet at a predetermined place in the hospital. Our instructor for the morning would then take us to see certain patients whom he had chosen for demonstration purposes. First the patient would be interviewed to find out what his problem was. Then he would be examined in order to demonstrate specific signs associated with his illness. This method of bedside teaching was one of the most important innovations in the education of medical students. It was initiated by Dr. William Osler, a Canadian physician.

As an example, we might see a patient who had hyperthyroidism (overactive thyroid gland). This condition is also known as toxic goitre. Many years ago it was called Graves Disease in honor of the physician who first described it. The symptoms of the patient (what he complained of) might consist of nervousness, excessive sweating, heat intolerance, palpitation, loss of weight and energy, increased appetite and shortness of breath. The signs (what you can see) demonstrated to the students might be warmness and moisture of the skin, a characteristic stare and protrusion of the eyeballs known as exophthalmos, enlargement of the thyroid gland (goitre), a fine tremor of the fingers and a very rapid heart rate. Over a period of two years, we would be fortunate to see hundreds of patients, many of them with rare conditions. Some of the patients who come to mind that were seen by our group had diseases which are not likely to be seen by today's medical students.

We saw a three-year old boy with diphtheria. He had a history of having a sore throat accompanied by a slight fever which had been present for a few hours. He then became quite lethargic and began to experience some difficulty with his breathing. With the assistance of the pediatrician who was caring for him, we were able to see the smooth, grey membrane which covered the back wall of the pharynx and extended onto both tonsils. The boy looked very sick.

Diphtheria is an infectious disease caused by a bacterium known as the Corynebacterium diphtheriae. This microorganism produces a powerful toxin which is responsible for many of the severe manifestations of the disease. Diphtheria is rarely seen today in Canada due to almost universal immunization against the disease. However, it is still prevalent in many developing countries. A safe and effective vaccine has been available since 1923.

It is important to make an accurate diagnosis of diphtheria so that antitoxin can be given promptly. Any delay increases the possibility of death. The antitoxin is effective in combating the effects of the toxin produced by the bacteria. Besides using the antitoxin, it is also important to give the patient adequate doses of penicillin in order to kill the bacteria. If the membrane extends to the larynx and causes obstruction, then immediate tracheotomy is needed. Diphtheria is 100% preventable by immunization of all infants with toxoid.

We saw a one-month old infant with a patent ductus arteriosus. The ductus arteriosus is a small artery which connects the pulmonary artery and the aorta. During fetal life and for a short period after birth, a large percentage of pulmonary arterial blood is shunted from the pulmonary artery to the aorta through this artery. Closure of the ductus arteriosus normally occurs a short time after the birth of the baby. If it remains patent (open), aortic blood is shunted into the pulmonary artery from the aorta. There are usually no symptoms associated with this condition initially, but the physical signs are striking. On placing a hand over the heart, a characteristic "thrill" (vibration) is felt. On listening to the heart with a stethoscope, a classic "murmur" (blowing sound) is heard which is usually described as "machinery-like murmur" because of its close resemblance to the sound of running machinery. Fortunately, even at that time (1948), surgical treatment was possible. The procedure consisted of opening the chest, identifying the ductus arteriosus, clamping it, tying it and cutting it. Open-heart surgery was not being done at that time because the heart-lung machine had not been developed, so there was no way of by-passing the heart. This development had to wait until the early 60s.

We saw an infant with rickets. Rickets is a metabolic disorder of growing bone which results in boney abnormalities. The disease is due to a deficiency of Vitamin D in the diet of the infant. This vitamin is essential to the regulation of the concentration of calcium and phosphorus in the blood. We were instructed to examine this infant for two signs of rickets, craniotabes and rachitic rosary. Craniotabes is detected by pressing firmly on the occipital (back) or parietal (side) area of the skull. A "ping-pong ball" sensation will be felt due to the thinning of the inner table of the skull. Rachitic rosary refers to the enlargement of the ribs which is felt (and sometimes seen) at the junction of the boney and cartilagenous regions of the ribs. These enlargements resemble small marbles. Since rickets is preventable by giving the infant adequate Vitamin D on a daily basis, it is very seldom seen in Canada today.

We saw a middle-aged man with active pulmonary tuberculosis. His history included fever, night sweats, weakness, productive (mucousy) cough and weight loss. When we examined his chest with our stethoscopes, we heard the characteristic rales (crackling sounds) of pneumonia. X-ray films of his chest revealed the characteristic area of consolidation (without air) of one lung. Tuberculosis was a common illness at the time that I attended university. As a matter of interest, the eldest son of our professor of medicine, Dr. John Scott, contracted tuberculosis when he was in his second year of medical school. He was required to drop out of school for over a year until the disease became inactive. Following this event, Dr. Scott had all of the medical students tested for tuberculosis with the tuberculin test and chest x-rays. Those who were tuberculin-negative were given BCG Vaccine to help boost their immunity to the disease. With better health care, nutrition and sanitation, tuberculosis has become rare. However, today, with widespread drug addiction and its associated malnutrition plus poor hygiene, the disease is once more beginning to manifest itself.

We saw a boy six years of age who had acute poliomyelitis. His initial history consisted of nausea, vomiting, diarrhea and fever (identical to many patients with influenza). However, it wasn't long before he developed signs suggestive of poliomyelitis-pain and spasms of the muscles of his legs followed by weakness of the muscles. A lumbar puncture (insertion of a needle into the spinal fluid) and examination of the cerebrospinal fluid revealed findings which were compatible with poliomyelitis.

Poliomyelitis (also called infantile paralysis) is an acute infection of the grey matter of the brain and spinal cord. It is caused by a specific virus. It is usually a disease of young children, but may at times affect infants and young adults. The virus is transmitted through the feces of an infected individual. The disease may present itself initially as a respiratory infection or an infection of the gastrointestinal tract. The patient may go on to manifest involvement of the nervous system by developing headache, stiffness of the neck, and paralysis of various muscles. When the cervical portion of the spinal cord is involved, there may be paralysis of the muscles of the shoulders, arms and neck. If the thoracic portion of the spinal cord is involved, there may be weakness of the muscles of the chest and upper abdomen. This may interfere somewhat with the patient's ability to breathe. Disease of the lumbar portion of the spinal cord produces weakness of the legs and muscles of the back and abdomen. When the brainstem is involved, the cranial nuclei are affected. The signs and symptoms will depend on which nuclei are involved. The muscles controlling the movement of the eyeballs may be affected or paralysis of the face might occur. There may be difficulty in swallowing and in speaking and difficulty in breathing. The symptoms and signs of poliomyelitis vary considerably and depend on which part of the nervous system is involved. Paralysis may be temporary or permanent. Fortunately, most patients infected with the virus recover completely.

We saw a number of patients with poliomyelitis. Some of them recovered completely, others developed paralyses of various muscles and a few required the use of a respirator (iron lung) in order to keep them alive.

In 1956, the Salk Vaccine was being used and by 1960 the Sabin Vaccine was available. This was given to the children on a cube of sugar. Since the development of these vaccines, poliomyelitis in Canada has been practically eliminated.

When I was in elementary school in Edmonton, I can recall the opening of schools in September being delayed because of an outbreak of poliomyelitis. At that time it was not known that the disease was caused by a virus, but since it was considered to be infectious, we were advised to avoid crowds. I had two close friends who had paralysis of their legs as a result of the disease.

At one of our bedside clinics, we saw a young boy with acute rheumatic fever. He had a history of recurrent sore throat, with accompanying fever. A few days prior to his admission to hospital, he began to develop pain in the knee and ankle joints. The pain migrated from one joint to another and was accompanied by swelling and decreased movement of the joint involved. He was admitted to hospital because he had developed a tachycardia (rapid heart rate) along with a heart murmur. We were seeing him in order to demonstrate the migratory arthritis and the murmur which indicated involvement of the mitral valve of the heart. This was referred to as rheumatic carditis.

Rheumatic fever is one of the complications of streptocccal infection of the throat. In the 1940s the illness was fairly common, but since the discovery and use of penicillin in treating streptococcal infections, the incidence of rheumatic fever has been reduced considerably.

As a matter of interest, two members of my class, Clarence Chouinard and Robert Paradny, had rheumatic fever when they were young. In both cases, the disease caused permanent damage to the heart valves. The damage to Clarence's heart was severe enough to require a valve replacement when he was in his sixties. He was well for many years after the surgery, but while attending a convention of radiologists in Australia, he flipped off an embolus (blood clot) from the artificial valve. The embolus lodged in the brain causing almost instant death.

Bob Paradny did not require heart surgery but he also died instantly. He was driving his car to the hospital where he did surgery in New York City when he was hit head-on by a truck, crushing him.

We were able to see patients who were in the various stages of syphilis. The first stage was demonstrated when we saw a young man in his early thirties with a chancre (papule) of the penis. Another young man was seen who presented with a generalized rash which resembled measles. However, the eruption was not due to measles, but represented the second stage of syphilis. I can recall seeing two patients with tertiary syphilis. The first one had involvement of the central nervous system, which resulted in a condition known as tabes dorsalis. In this condition, the posterior columns of the spinal cord are affected. When this occurs, the sensation of the soles of the feet is lost causing the so-called tabetic gait. When walking, the feet are held wide apart, they are lifted high in the air and stomped forcefully to the ground.

One of the most striking patients I have ever seen was in the third stage of cardiovascular syphilis. This type involves the larger arteries of the body. Small arteries, called the vasa vasorum, supply blood to the walls of the large arteries. With syphilis, an inflammatory reaction occurs in the vasa vasorum causing obstruction of these arteries. This results in damage to the elastic tissue of the wall of the large artery. When the damage is severe enough, the wall weakens, then bulges, producing what is known as an aneurysm. This patient had a large aneurysm of the arch of the aorta, located just after the artery leaves the heart. When we saw this patient, he was sitting up in bed. As we looked at him, his whole chest wall pulsated with each contraction of the heart. It was an amazing thing to witness. At that time, there was no possible treatment available for this condition. The aneurysm would ultimately rupture causing almost instantaneous death due to exsanguination (severe loss of blood).

In our pathology lectures, a good deal of time was devoted to the discussion of syphilis in its various forms. Syphilis is a chronic systemic infection caused by the spirochaete (a coil-shaped microorganism) Treponema pallidum. It is usually sexually transmitted and is characterized by an incubation period averaging three weeks, followed by a primary lesion, the chancre. The chancre is painless, infectious, and disappears spontaneously. This is followed by the secondary stage in which the skin and mucous membranes are involved with the appearance of skin eruptions of various types along with general enlargement of the lymph nodes. These lesions also clear spontaneously without treatment. The patient then goes through a latent period of subclinical infection lasting many years. In about 40% of cases, a tertiary stage occurs characterized by progressive destruction of the cardiovascular and nervous systems. There was no known cure for syphilis until 1943 when penicillin was used to treat this condition for the first time.

Since the Treponema pallidum is capable of attacking all of the cells and organs of the body, syphilis was given the name "the Great Imitator". The symptoms and signs of syphilitic infections could mimic those of many other diseases.

At the time that I was in medical school (1945-1949), there were really only two venereal diseases of significance, gonorrhea and syphilis. The term "venereal" is derived from Venus, the Greek goddess of love. The term "venereal" is no longer used. Instead, the term "sexually-transmitted diseases" (STD) is used. The list of sexually-transmitted diseases has become longer and now includes trichomonas, herpes simplex, hepatitis B and C, Human Immunodeficiency Virus (HIV), which causes Acquired Immunodeficiency Syndrome, more commonly referred to as AIDS, and chlamydia. Today, the most common STD is chlamydia infection.

When I was in the third year of medical school, I awakened one morning, turned over in bed, and experienced a sudden, severe, sharp pain in my neck. The muscles of my neck went into spasm immediately. The pain and spasm were so severe that I was unable to hold my head up straight. Fortunately for me, my first clinic at the University Hospital was with Dr. Rostrop, associate professor of Orthopedics. As soon as he saw me, he asked me why I wasn't holding my head up. When I explained what had happened, he examined me and sent me to have x-rays of the neck. The x-rays showed that I had dislocated a couple of the apophyseal joints of the cervical vertebrae.

That evening, under general anaesthesia, Dr. Rostrop reduced the dislocations. When I awoke, my neck was immobilized in a cervical collar. I wore this collar continually for the next eight weeks. Although it made studying and other activities a little more difficult, it corrected the problem. I have been thankful for the prompt care given to me by Dr. Rostrop as I have not had any trouble with my neck since this one episode.

During the third and fourth years of medical school, our afternoons were filled with lectures. From 1:00 P.M. until 5:00 P.M., lectures were given by the professors of the various departments of medicine, surgery, pediatrics, obstetrics and gynecology, ophthalmology, otolaryngology and orthopedics. We also had lectures and labs in pathology.

Pathology is the science which deals with the changes that occur in cells as a result of injury or disease. It is probably the most important subject taught in medical school. The textbook used by us was written by William Boyd. This book was a real pleasure to read. It was almost like reading a first-class novel. One of the many quotations of Boyd will always stick in my mind. After doing thousands of autopsies on patients who had died from innumerable conditions he said *"I am not surprised that these people have died. What does surprise me is that so many of them were able to live so long with so much pathology"*.

In the third year of medical school, we had a short course in surgical pathology. This course was given on Saturday mornings by one of the professors of pathology. He was a rather eccentric person and was inclined to say and do things which were designed to shock the students. He would bring specimens which had been removed during various surgical procedures into the classroom, demonstrate the characteristics of the specimens, and then briefly discuss the disease which had necessitated the surgery.

One morning, he began his class by remarking *"Today's medical students never seem to get syphilis"*. This seemed to imply that there was something lacking in the students he was teaching. On one of his morning sessions, he walked into the classroom carrying a tray on which there was a huge specimen. He put the tray on the table in front of the classroom, picked up the specimen in his two hands, held it out in front of him at arm's length and let it drop to the floor. There was a loud "thud" as the specimen hit the floor. He then proceeded to tell us that this specimen was the liver which had been removed from a patient during autopsy. The patient had died from cirrhosis produced by indulging in large quantities of alcohol. The alcohol had acted like a poison and had gradually destroyed the liver cells, which had been replaced by fibrous tissue (scar tissue). The condition was therefore given the name "alcoholic cirrhosis". He handed the specimen to one of the students in the classroom who, after examining it closely, passed it on to the student beside him. When it was my turn to examine the organ, I couldn't help comparing it to a large, firm, rubber ball.

On another occasion, this same professor rushed into the classroom carrying a large tray overflowing with specimens. The specimens turned

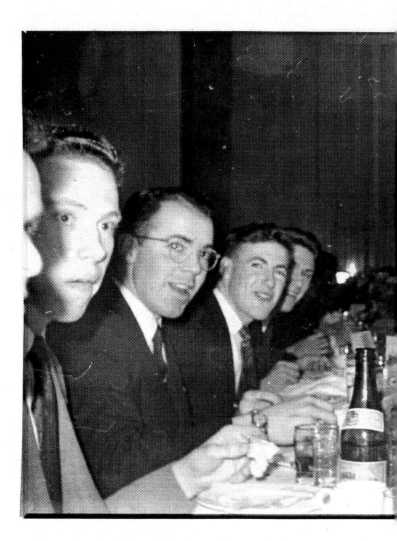

PHOTO 18 [Photo of graduation dinner, Mac-Donald Hotel, 1949. Author is second from front on right]

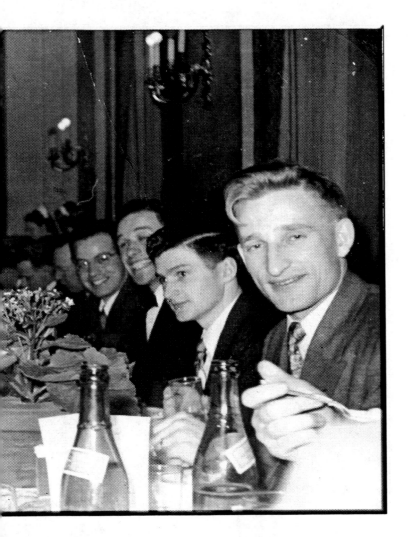

out to be appendices which had been removed at various stages of inflammation. Some appeared almost normal while others were gangrenous or had ruptured. He quickly placed the tray on the table in front of the classroom and rushed out to get some

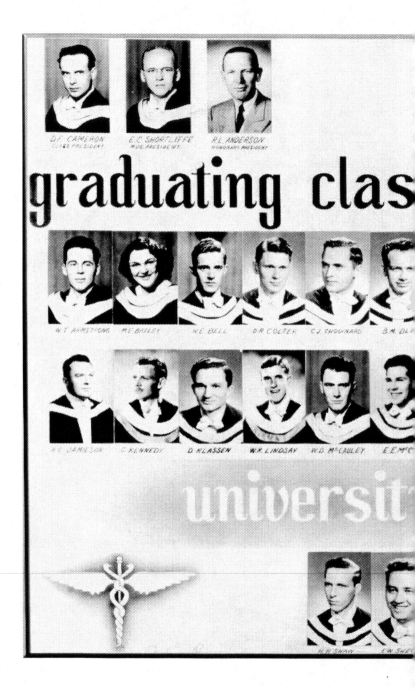

PHOTO 19 [Photo of author's graduating class]

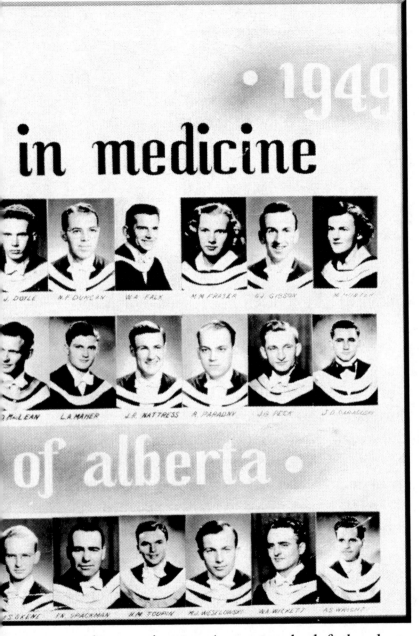

in medicine

1949

of alberta

J. DOYLE   N.F. DUNCAN   W.A. FALK   M.M. FRASER   G.J. GIBSON   H. HUNTER

MacLEAN   L.R. MAHER   J.R. NATTRESS   R. PARADNY   J.G. PECK   J.O. RAWLISON

S. SKENE   F.N. SPACKMAN   H.M. TODRIN   M.J. WESILOWSKI   W.A. WICKETT   A.S. WRIGHT

other specimens. As soon as he left the classroom, one of the students bolted for the door. He returned within a minute or two, before the professor had

69

returned, and carefully placed a specimen on the very top of all the other specimens so that it stuck out like a sore thumb.

When the professor returned, he placed another tray full of specimens on the table, then picked up the first tray he had brought into the room. Immediately a strange look appeared on his face. He didn't say a word but proceeded to pass the tray to one of the students in the front. When the tray reached me, I was amazed to find that the specimen at the top of the appendices was a penis! I realized then that the student had rushed to the anatomy lab, sliced the penis off one of the cadavers and put it on top of the specimens of appendices.

Writing about pathology reminds me of the small museum which was located on the second floor of the medical building just outside of the anatomy lab. This museum contained dozens of unusual specimens which had been collected by the departments of anatomy and pathology over a period of many years. The specimens had been placed in glass jars filled with formaldehyde in order to preserve them. The jars were in glass cabinets. The specimen which always caught my eye as I walked past these cabinets was that of the full head of a man. He had apparently decided that life wasn't worth living, had placed a shotgun into his mouth and pulled the trigger. There was a huge hole, about three inches in diameter, where the top of the skull had been blown away.

On the television news, we are forever being told about people being involved in motor vehicle accidents. When a person has been killed in one of these accidents, the reporter never fails to advise us that death was "instantaneous". How he has been able to be so positive of this has always been a mystery to me. In the case of the man whose head was in the jar, I think I can safely say that death was "instantaneous".

As I look back over my life, I realize how fortunate I was to have been able to obtain an education in medicine. From the time of fertilization of the ovum by the spermatazoon, through the stages of development of the fetus, to the miracle of birth, the human journey is a fascinating one. We continue with the development of the infant and young child, through adolescence and ultimately adulthood. After studying the changes which occur during normal development, we went on to study the changes brought about by abnormalities of growth, injuries and disease. Learning how to treat these pathologies was an entirely new and exciting area of study.

Over the years, I've had many people say to me   "*I could never have been a doctor because*:
"*I can't stand the sight of blood*"; or
"*I could never cut into someone*"; or
"*I wouldn't be able to tolerate seeing some one in severe pain*"; or
"*I couldn't stand to watch someone die*".

My answer to this is usually *"Over a period of time, a person can get used to almost anything"*.

I must confess, that all through medical school and internship, I do not recall being disturbed by anything that I saw. However, I do recall the odd time when a classmate might have been a bit squeamish.

I can recall one incident in particular which makes me smile whenever I think of it. One of the members of our group of six had a tendency to rush ahead of the rest of us in order to get to see the patient first. On this particular occasion, we were going to see a patient who was in a private room. As was usual, this particular student rushed into the room quickly ahead of anyone else. Before the rest of us had even passed through the door, he made a 180° turn and was quickly heading back out of the room. What he had encountered was a patient who had a resection of the large intestine for cancer. The nurse had removed the dressing of the patient to expose a colostomy (the opening of the large intestine onto the surface of the body) for our observation. Since we had not been advised beforehand what we were going to witness, the site of the opening of the colostomy apparently was quite a shock to the student. After that episode, he was a little more cautious about being the first one at the bedside of the patient.

CHAPTER 6: JUNIOR INTERNSHIP

Getting Closer To The Real Action

It is much easier to stay out of trouble than it is to get out of trouble.
Lyon H. Appleby M.D. - 1950 -
Head, Department of Surgery
St. Paul's Hospital, Vancouver, B.C.

On May 20, 1949, the day that I had just finished writing my last final examination, I was having dinner with my girlfriend, Connie Eccles, in her apartment when there was a knock at the door. I opened the door to find Mrs. Vi Passmore standing there. Vi was a neighbour of Mr. and Mrs. Laurie Fee with whom I boarded during the last two years of medical school.

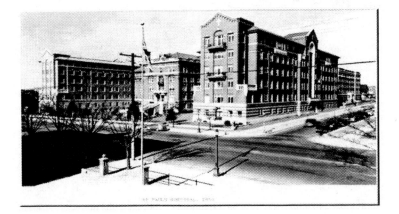

PHOTO 20 [Photo of St. Paul's Hospital as it appeared during author's period of internship]

Vi informed me that my mother had just phoned her from Vancouver to advise that my grandmother had just passed away in St. Paul's Hospital. This was a sad moment for me as I had always been close to my grandmother. My mother requested that I take the next train from Edmonton to Vancouver in order that I might attend the funeral. My grandmother had died of congestive heart failure. She had been in hospital for several days, but my mother did

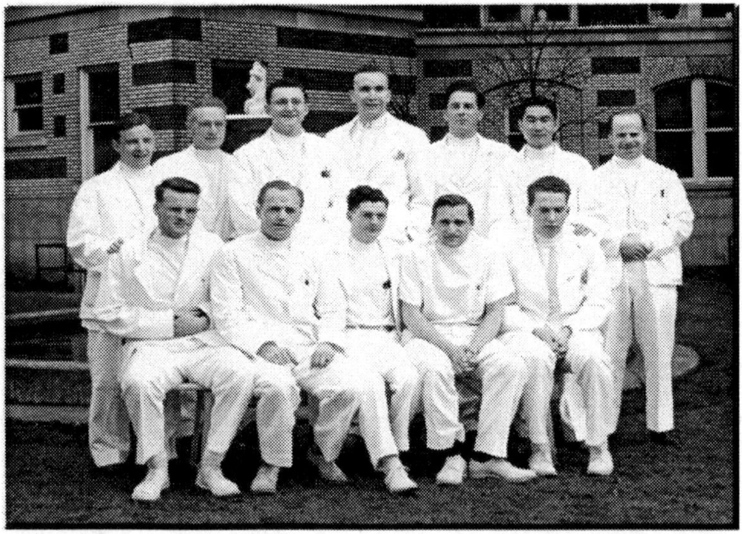

PHOTO 21 [Interns – St. Paul's Hospital, Vancouver – 1950]

Front row – 3rd from left – author
4th from left – Dr. Chouinard
Far right – Dr. Doyle
Back row - 3rd from left – Dr. Ragan
5th from left – Dr. Armstrong
6th from left – Dr. Chou]

not let me know for fear that the news would interfere with my studying. Apparently my grandmother
had told other patients in her room that her grandson
would be starting to intern at St. Paul's in July, but
they thought she was just a raving old woman.

I attended my grandmother's funeral,
remained in Vancouver for a few days and then
returned to Edmonton to attend the graduation cere-
monies. It was a very exciting day for all of us. I
was twenty-four at the time. Four of my classmates
were only twenty-two. It's not likely that students
will ever again graduate from medical school while
in their early twenties.

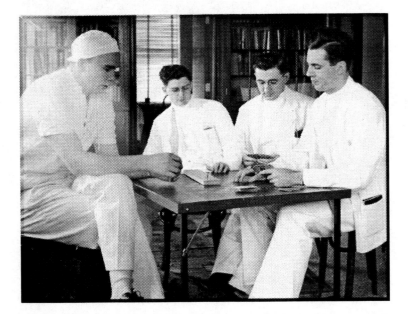

**PHOTO 22 [Relaxing at St. Paul's - Author 2nd
from left]**

I would like to point out that there appears to be a common misconception among the public (and surprisingly among some members of the medical and nursing professions) that part of the graduation ceremony of medical students consists in taking the Oath of Hippocrates.

When I graduated from the University of Alberta in 1949, I did not take the Hippo-cratic Oath, nor any other oath for that matter. Anyone who is familiar with this oath should realize that it is contrary to the teachings of the Catholic, Jewish and Islamic religions to swear by any of the pagan gods.

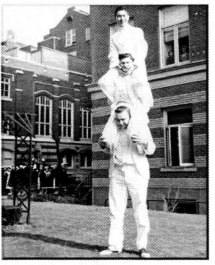

PHOTO 23 [Goofing it up - Author in centre]

It is perhaps worth noting that Hippocrates, a Greek physician who lived in the fifth century B.C. and who has been given the name " *Father of Medicine* ", was not in favor of abortions nor euthanasia. Both of these are accepted by many physicians today. The oath is reproduced on page 95.

The year that I graduated was the first year that graduates of medicine from the University of

Alberta were permitted to intern outside of Edmonton. Five of us made arrangements to do our internship at St. Paul's Hospital in Vancouver; Pat Doyle, Bill Armstrong, John Ragan, Clarence Chouinard and me. Three classmates went to the Vancouver General, two went to Victoria, one went to New York City, one to Los Angeles and several stayed in Edmonton.

We began our internship on July 1, 1949, and were to spend the next twelve months practically living in St. Paul's Hospital. At that time, the living quarters for the interns were situated on the southwest corner of the first floor of the hospital. There were two interns to a room, shower facilities and a large common room for relaxation. Hospital clothes and meals were supplied and we had our own private dining room with very good food. We were paid the princely sum of seventy-five dollars per month. At first, we did not think too highly of this rate of pay, but when we learned that our classmates at the General were receiving twenty-five dollars per month, we felt much better about it.

There were twelve junior interns at the hospital, and all of us were recent graduates. Five of us were from Edmonton and the remaining seven were from various parts of Canada. Since there was no medical school in British Columbia at that time, there were no graduates from B.C. The medical school at the University of British Columbia did not start its first class until 1950. As there were no senior interns and only one resident at St. Paul's, all of the work was done by the twelve junior interns. This proved to be an excellent choice for us as we got an enormous amount of practical experience during the year.

For purposes of training, the program was divided into twelve areas. These consisted of surgery A, B and C, medicine A, B and C, pediatrics, orthopedics, obstetrics and gynecology, anaesthesia, radiology and the Indian and Marine service. Each intern spent one month on each of these services.

While on the surgery service, we were expected to see each patient the day before surgery, complete a history and physical examination, assist at surgery the following day and be responsible for the post-operative care of the patients. Surgery began at 8 A.M. each weekday and finished around 4 P.M. Since the intern was always the first assistant, he got a good view of everything that went on during the surgical procedure.

Dr. Lyon Appleby Sr. was the head of the department of surgery and also in charge of Surgery A. He did a tremendous volume of surgery every week day. It was not unusual for him to do a gastrectomy (removal of the stomach), cholecystectomy (removal of the gallbladder), a large bowel resection and an inguinal hernia in one day. He was a master technician and worked very quickly. He never seemed to get into trouble during a surgical procedure. Instead of wearing the usual head-covering that everyone else did while in the operating room, he wore his own special little blue cap. After completing surgery, he would remove his cap, fold it and tuck it into the top of his O.R. pants. He also did not wear the ordinary clothes supplied by the hospital to be used while in the operating room, but wore his own clothes made of seersucker because the material was lighter and cooler. As far as the nursing sisters were concerned, Dr. Appleby could do no wrong.

Prior to spending the month on Dr. Appleby's service, the intern was briefed by the one leaving his service as to what was expected of him. Dr. Appleby demanded that all of his patients were to be asleep by the time they reached the operating room. This meant that the intern would have to prepare a mixture of sodium amytal to be given intravenously to the patient after he had been transferred from his bed to a stretcher. The intern would then have to accompany the patient from his room into the elevator and to the operating room – and he'd better not be late getting to the O.R. Dr. Appleby was so quick at doing his surgical procedures that one day he had completed doing one hernia on a patient and was starting a second one when I arrived in the operating room fifteen minutes late. Needless to say, he wasn't pleased with me.

The head of the department of anaesthesia, Dr. Roche, gave all of the anaesthetics for Dr. Appleby. He did not give any anaesthetics for any of the other surgeons. Dr. Appleby also had his own personal operating room nurse, Molly Smith, who assisted him with every surgical procedure. She knew which instrument he needed before he even asked for it. He would merely hold out his right hand and Molly would slap the instrument into his palm. It was an amazing thing to witness. Molly was personally hired by Dr. Appleby, who paid her salary. Dr. Appleby also had his own nurse, Mary Gallagher, who looked after all of the post-operative care of his patients. I don't think he ever saw a patient after the surgery was completed. The interns were not allowed to write any post-op orders for his patients.

The intern had very little to do during the surgical procedures. His main job was to hold the retractors so that Dr. Appleby could see the surgical field properly, and to cut the sutures. Dr. Appleby always tied three knots and the intern was to cut the suture right at the third knot. He used to say that Forest Lawn Cemetery was filled with interns who had cut the sutures too long. He was usually very quiet when he was operating and did not usually volunteer any information unless he was asked a specific question. However, he did have a number of pearls of wisdom for the intern on his service, such as:

"It is easier to stay out of trouble than to get out of trouble"; and

"Surgery in the absence of pathology (disease) *is a cinch"*.

This last was a reference to those surgeons who were in the habit of removing "normal" organs, such as the appendix or the gallbladder.

In all honesty, I can't say that I enjoyed my month with Dr. Appleby because I always felt a certain amount of stress when I was assisting him. I somehow had the feeling that he really didn't need me to help him and that I was in his way most of the time.

In contrast to Dr. Appleby, the head of Surgery B service, Dr. B.T.H. Marteinsson, was very easy going. He went out of his way to explain to the intern what he was doing and why he was doing it. He worked very slowly and methodically. He was also an excellent surgeon. I was quite relaxed whenever I assisted him with surgery and had a feeling that he appreciated my help.

Most of the surgeons were easy to get along with and went out of their way to instruct us. However, as in any field of endeavour, there is always the one who is unpleasant. One surgeon in particular never ceased to be dissatisfied with the way the sutures were cut by the intern. Nothing seemed to satisfy him. Bill Armstrong, one of the interns who never took any nonsense from anyone, decided to get even with this man one morning while he was assisting at surgery. The first suture he cut too long on purpose. Of course, the surgeon remarked "*Too long*". The next suture, Bill purposely cut too short. The surgeon bellowed "*Too short*". After the surgeon finished tying the third suture, Bill purposely cut the knot right off. The surgeon didn't say a word for the rest of the morning.

On another occasion, when Bill was assisting the same surgeon and forever being raked over the coals for not doing things to the liking of the surgeon, he finally got fed up with the abuse. He stepped back from the operating table, removed his gloves and said to the surgeon *"I guess you don't need me anymore"*. With that, he walked out of the operating room. Apparently, after that episode, the surgeon treated Bill with a little more respect – at least for a few days.

It was not unusual in those days, (when the surgeon was God in the operating room) for him to rap an assistant on the knuckles with a forceps or other instrument in order to show his displeasure. One day this same surgeon struck Bill on the knuckles for doing something he didn't like. To the surgeon's amazement, Bill picked up a forceps and rapped the surgeon back. Such an act was unheard of in those days, but Bill apparently got away with it.

My three months on the medical service were very rewarding. I became more knowledgeable in the diagnosis and treatment of conditions such as heart attacks, pneumonia, hypertension, diabetes, peptic ulcer, stroke and many other diseases. It didn't take us long to learn who were the good internists and who were not worth wasting our time with. The best internist at the hospital without a doubt was Dr. W.H.B. (Bill) Hurlburt. I always made a point of being at the nursing station on two West of the hospital early every morning because I knew that he would start there to make his rounds to see his patients. It was a great opportunity to talk to him about his patients, to ask him questions and to pick his brain on any medical subject.

It was a real learning experience to be asked to accompany him when he had been requested to do a consultation on a patient by another doctor. He did the most thorough history and physical examination of any doctor I have ever known. He spent at least an hour with the patient whenever he did a consultation. In those days, internists were relatively poorly paid compared to surgeons, but this didn't have any effect on the time he spent with the patient. If there was a tough diagnosis to be made, Dr. Hurlburt could usually be counted on to make it.

During our month on pediatrics, we became more at ease in examining infants and young children. Examining these tiny patients is an art which requires gentleness and patience. Some doctors never acquire this. You have to like children and be at ease with them. You must never cause them any pain unnecessarily as they will never forget it and never forgive you.

During my month on pediatrics, I experienced one of the most heart-rending situations in my career. One evening I was called to the pediatric ward by the head nurse. There was a five-year old boy who had been on the ward for a number of days and who had tuberculous meningitis. This condition was invariably fatal and the boy had just died. His mother was with him at the time of his death and she refused to let the nurse take him to the morgue. She thought it would be too cold and lonely for him there. The nurse asked me to speak to the mother and try to persuade her to change her mind. I spoke to the mother for some time and managed to get her to agree to remain with her son for one more hour and then to allow the nurse to take him to the morgue. The mother was a widow in her late thirties and this was her only child. This tragedy still comes to my mind on occasion in spite of the fact that it has been fifty years since it happened.

When I look back now after all of these years, I believe the month that I spent on the orthopedic service was the most enjoyable of all. Dr. A.S. McConkey was the chief of orthopedics and went out of his way to teach the interns. He had taken his orthopedic training in England and had spent some of his training period working under one of the most renowned orthopedists of that time – Sir Reginald Watson-Jones. As a result, he was a very capable surgeon.

Dr. McConkey was always in a happy mood when he was operating. At the time that I was on his service, there was a very popular tune which he sang every morning at the beginning of surgery – "I've Got A Lovely Bunch Of Coconuts". Of course, everyone in the O.R. couldn't help but join him in the singing. It was a very pleasant way to begin the day.

At that time, the major fear in doing surgery on the bones and joints was the possibility of introducing infection, which might result in the loss of a limb or even a life. While we were on this service, we were required to wear two face masks, and we did not remove our surgical gloves immediately after completing a surgical procedure, but waited until we were ready to scrub for the next case. The "business ends" of the surgical instruments were never touched by our hands, but were always handled with sterile instruments. This was the so-called Lane's No-touch Technique. Patients were admitted to hospital two days before the surgery date so that a very careful and thorough prep of the skin of the operative area could be carried out. At that time, amputation of the lower extremity because of gangrene due to faulty circulation to the limb was a fairly common procedure. One morning, while we were preparing to do an amputation, Dr. McConkey remarked *"We can do a lot of things in orthopedic surgery, but we can't replace blood vessels"*. It would be a number of years before major blood vessels could be replaced with synthetic grafts thereby reducing considerably the number of amputations required due to deficiency of the circulation.

One morning while I was assisting Dr. McConkey with a fusion of the spine we got into the discussion of back pain and its causes. I mentioned that I had never really been shown in medical school how to examine a person's back properly. On hearing this, he invited me to come over to his office the following afternoon after I had finished my hospital work and he would show me how to examine a back properly. I took him up on his offer and appeared at his office at 3:00 P.M. the following day. He told me that I had arrived just at the right time as he had just seen a young man with chronic back pain and was waiting for him to undress so that he could examine him. We went into the examining room together and he introduced me to the patient, telling him that I was a young doctor who was anxious to learn how to examine patients who had back problems. He then proceeded to show me in detail how to carry out a thorough examination of the patient. It was a lesson I never forgot.

Dr. McConkey admitted many patients to hospital with interesting, unusual and sometimes rare conditions. There was one of his patients in particular who will always remain in my memory. He was five years old. This young boy had a condition known as osteogenesis imperfecta, also called fragilitis ossium, but most often referred to as brittle bone disease. He had sustained a fracture of the tibia, an injury, which required treatment. He had been in hospital many times before for the treatment of innumerable fractures usually involving the arms or legs. He was very small for his age. His head was large for the size of his body. His arms and legs were severely bowed as a result of fractures healing in malposition. He could not stand and was unable to sit up without assistance. In spite of his severe disability, he was surprisingly cheerful and talkative.

Osteogenesis imperfecta is a congenital condition in which there is an abnormal development of the bones. It is actually a type of osteoporosis in which there is marked thinning of the outer layer (the cortex) of the bone and a decrease in the amount of calcium in the medulla (the centre) of the bone. This makes the person susceptible to multiple fractures from simple injuries. There is no treatment for this condition other than to try as much as possible to prevent fractures from occurring and to treat them promptly when they do occur.

The month I spent on the obstetrical and gynecological service was exhausting. I was required to do a history and physical examination on every patient admitted to the service and to be present in the case room for every delivery. This meant that I was unable to leave the hospital for the whole month unless I could persuade one of the other interns to fill in for me for a few hours. This didn't happen very often. During the month, I was first assistant at many gynecological surgical procedures and became familiar with all of the more common operations. Although I was allowed to do a few normal deliveries in the case room and to sew up a few episiotomies (an incision made into the vagina in order to enlarge the opening at the time of delivering a baby), I did not have the opportunity to learn many of the things I would need to know in order to practise good obstetrics.

During the month on anaesthesia I learned the basics of using local anaesthesia, spinal anaesthesia and the principles of general anaesthesia. I did not get enough experience in giving general anaesthetics to be really comfortable with this by the time that I had completed my month.

The Indian and Marine service was a very valuable service for us. Dr. Pinkerton had a contract to look after all of the men in the merchant marine service who visited Vancouver. If they required any surgery they were admitted to St. Paul's Hospital. Dr. Pinkerton was very generous in allowing the interns to do some of the surgical procedures. Many a hernia and appendectomy were carried out while the intern was on this service.

Dr. Waddington had a similar contract to look after the Indians who were admitted to St. Paul's Hospital. He also allowed the interns to do quite a bit of surgery. We were all very appreciative of the experience we had gained during the month spent on the Indian and Marine service.

There were two other duties which were allotted to the interns. One of us was always scheduled to be on call to the emergency room for anyone who might happen to appear there. Another intern was always on call to see any patients in the hospital if a nurse felt it was necessary. We called this "House Call".

The first day that I was on house call, I was called to the third floor of the hospital to see a patient who had just recently returned from surgery. He was an adult male, had just had his tonsils removed and had started to bleed. At that stage of my training, I had never seen a tonsillectomy and had no idea how to deal with post-operative bleeding following this procedure.

However, as happened many times during my year of internship, the head nurse came to my rescue. She had everything set up to deal with the situation. The patient was one of Dr. Grimett's, an otolaryngologist. The nurse proceeded to advise me how Dr. Grimett handled post-operative bleeding and guided me through the routine. In spite of her excellent instructions, I was not able to get the bleeding under control and had to make arrangements for the patient to return to the operating room in order to get the bleeding stopped. What an introduction to "House Call" that turned out to be.

One never knew what to expect when called to see a patient, but in time we became more knowledgeable, more confident and less timid in handling emergency situations. Often, during these emergencies, I thought of a lecture given by Dr. William Osler to medical students. The title of the lecture was "Equanimitas". Osler defined Equanimitas as the ability to stay calm in the face of disaster. He believed that every doctor must possess this ability. With this, I would heartily agree.

One evening when I was on call to the emergency room, I was called to see a man who had severed several of the tendons in his hand while using a knife to cut meat. I phoned the orthopedic surgeon who was on call and advised him of the problem. He told me to make arrangements to take the patient to surgery in order to repair the tendons and that he would come right down to the hospital. I was in the operating room, scrubbed and gowned, when the surgeon appeared at the doorway of the O.R. He told me to go ahead and start repairing the tendons. When I advised him that I not only had never repaired a tendon, but had never seen one repaired, he said he would explain things to me as we went along. And so, with the help of the nurse, and with the orthopod looking over my shoulder, I carried out my first surgical procedure.

During my periods on call to the emergency room, I quickly learned how to handle many of the less difficult situations, such as the removal of a foreign body from the eye, the suturing of wounds, dressing of burns, treatment of nosebleeds and fractured noses and many, many other procedures. The first baby I ever delivered was in a taxi just outside of the door of the emergency room. At the time it appeared to be quite an emergency. However, anyone who has done any amount of obstetrics knows that the ones to worry about are not those who deliver spontaneously and precipitously, but the ones who require assistance with the delivery.

Speaking about the delivery of a baby reminds me of one, four days old, who was admitted to the pediatric service with an unusual infection. On examination, there was a copious, thick, creamy discharge present in both eyes. The eyelids and conjunctivae were red and swollen. Laboratory examination of the discharge revealed the bacterial organisms Neisseria gonorrhea, thus confirming the provisional diagnosis of gonococcal conjunctivitis (ophthalmia neonatorium). The infection was treated with penicillin injections, cleansing the eyes with cotton soaked in normal saline followed by the instillation of aureomycin eyedrops. The response to treatment was good with rapid clearing of the infection over a period of a few days.

Gonococcal infection of the eyes of a newborn was not common. After the delivery of an infant in hospital, a drop of 1% silver nitrate was instilled into each eye followed by irrigation of the eyes with normal saline. This was done before the infant left the delivery room to be taken to the nursery. The silver nitrate caused desquamation of the superficial layer of the cornea. In the event that the baby had been exposed to the gonococcal bacteria during its passage through the birth canal, any infected tissue was removed. This infant had been delivered at home, had passed through an infected birth canal, had not been treated prophylactically with silver nitrate and therefore became infected. Since silver nitrate is very irritating to the cornea, causing a chemical irritation, sometimes followed by bacterial infection, this form of prophylaxis has been replaced by the use of aureomycin or tetracycline eye drops. Today, the treatment of choice for this type of infection is the antibiotic ceftriaxon, given daily for seven days plus irrigation of the eyes every thirty minutes with normal saline.

I was having a late dinner in the private dining room for the interns one evening when the telephone rang. I answered the phone to find that the caller was the head nurse of the premature nursery. A newborn infant had just been admitted to the nursery and the nurse wanted me to see the infant. Being young and eager, I went immediately and was amazed at what greeted me there. A full-term, male infant was in one of the incubators. Except for the fact that his abdomen was covered with a sheet of plastic, he looked like any normal infant. However, when the nurse removed the plastic covering and underlying gauze, I was stunned at what I saw. The infant had what is known as an eventration of the abdomen. A large part of the abdominal wall was missing and loops of bowel were lying in the open for me to see. The liver and spleen were also plainly visible. Early in fetal life, the small intestine lies outside of the abdominal cavity. By the tenth week of development, the intestine returns into the abdomen and the abdominal wall closes over it. For some unknown reason, closure had failed to occur in this infant. Eventration of the abdomen is very rare. It requires early surgical treatment.

While awaiting surgery, a number of things needed to be attended to.

A nasogastric tube was passed into the stomach in order to decrease accumulation of air in the bowel. A cutdown was done so that intravenous fluids could be given continuously. The intestines needed to be kept moist by wrapping them in gauze sponges that had been soaked in warm normal saline solution. A plastic sheet was wrapped around the defect to limit water and heat loss. Broad-spectrum antibiotics were given intravenously in order to help prevent infection. Within a few hours of birth, the infant was taken to surgery. Dr. Marteinsson, one of the very capable general surgeons at St. Paul's Hospital, managed to free the skin of the abdominal wall sufficiently so that closure of the defect was possible. At a later date, the abdominal wall was strengthened by utilizing available muscles and fascia along with sheets of synthetic material. The infant remained in hospital for a number of weeks surviving several surgical procedures. I had the privilege of assisting with his pre-operative and post-operative care.

As a matter of interest, during the month I spent on the surgical service of Dr. Marteinsson (Surgery B), I was assisting him late one evening with a patient who had a bowel obstruction. While he was carefully freeing the adhesions which were causing the obstruction, in my enthusiasm to help him, I exerted a little too much tension on the bowel causing it to split in two. Most surgeons would have become pretty upset with such a mishap. However, Dr. Marteinsson, in his usually calm and quiet way, merely said *"I guess you know now how much traction you can exert on the bowel before it tears"*.

Early in this chapter, I mentioned that there were twelve junior interns, no senior interns and only one resident at St. Paul's Hospital when I began my internship in July of 1949. (A resident refers to a doctor who has graduated with a medical degree, following which he embarks on a four or five year training program in one of the specialties.) The one resident at the hospital was Dr. Ying Chou. Dr. Chou was the resident on the pediatric service. He had been born and raised in Canton, China. He was the oldest child in a large family. His father was a doctor, as were several of his siblings.

Ying had been sent from China to the Hospital for Sick Children in Toronto in order to take his training. After spending two years at Sick Children's, he decided to complete his training in Vancouver at St. Paul's Hospital. He was therefore in the third year of his training program when I began my internship. His presence at St. Paul's was extremely fortunate for me and the other interns.

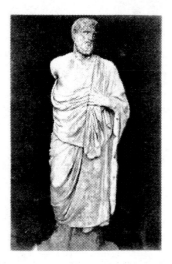

Hippocrates, statue Hippocrates (460-377 BC)

PHOTO 24 [PHOTO OF HIPPOCRATES]

Ying was a very hard-working, serious, and devoted resident. His command of the English language was very good. He went out of his way to teach the interns while they were on the pediatric service. Most of what I know about the care of infants and children I owe to Dr. Chou.

When he had completed his training and passed the examinations, he remained in Vancouver where he practised for many years. Because of him, I felt confident in treating infants and children when I left St. Paul's and started country practice in Quesnel.

PHYSICIAN'S OATH

I swear by Apollo the physician, by Aesculapius, Hygeia, and Panacea, and I take to witness all the gods, all the goddesses, to keep according to my ability and my judgment the following Oath:

To consider dear to me as my parents him who taught me this art; to live in common with him and if necessary to share my goods with him; to look upon his children as my own brothers, to teach them this art if they so desire without fee or written promise; to impart to my sons and the sons of the master who taught me and the disciples who have enrolled themselves and have agreed to the rules of the profession, but to these alone, the precepts and the instruction. I will prescribe regimen for the good of my patients according to my ability and my judgment and never do harm to anyone. To please no one will I prescribe a deadly drug, nor give advices which may cause his death. Nor will I give a woman a pessary to procure abortion. But I will preserve the purity of my life and my heart. I will not cut for stone, even for patients in whom the disease is manifest; I will leave this operation to be performed by practitioners (specialists in this art). In every house where I come I will enter only for the good of my patients, keeping myself far from all intentional ill-doing and all seduction, and especially from the pleasure of love with women or with men, be they free or slaves. All that may come to my knowledge in the exercise of my profession or outside of my profession or in daily commerce with men, which ought not to be spread abroad, I will keep secret and will never reveal. If I keep this oath faithfully, may I enjoy my life and practice my art, respected by all men and in all times, but if I swerve from it or violate it, may the reverse be my lot.

\- HIPPOCRATES

PHOTO 25
[COPY OF HIPPOCRATES' OATH]

CHAPTER 7: SENIOR INTERNSHIP

Lots of Experience

*Breast milk is for babies; Cow's milk is for calves.
Breast milk is best because it doesn't have to be
warmed, you can take it on picnics,
the cat can't get at it, and it comes in such cute containers.*

*Allan Brown, Head Physician at the Toronto's
Hospital for Sick Children – 1994*

At the completion of internship, it was customary for the interns to carry on into general practice or to continue on into a four-year residency program in one of the specialties. Instead of doing either of these, four of us decided to stay on at St. Paul's Hospital for a second year of training. Pat Doyle and I would take six months of pediatrics and six months of medicine. Clarence Chouinard and Bob McNaughton would take six months of surgery and six months of obstetrics.

Before I started my second year, I took my one-week vacation and went back to Edmonton where Connie and I were married. We then took a few days to make our way back to Vancouver, stopping at Jasper for three days. While at Jasper, we decided to take a boat trip to Maligne Lake. When the owner of the boat, Rainbow Jack, learned that we had just been married, he said that the trip would be

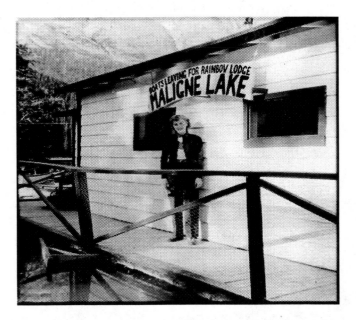

PHOTO 26 [Author's wife at the dock, Maligne Lake]

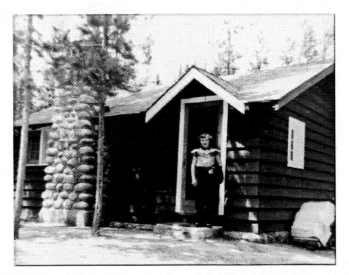

PHOTO 27 [The log cabin in Jasper where author and wife spent the first night of married life]

free - a wedding present from him to us. We also stopped at Lake Louise and Banff for one day. The honeymoon was very short, but a welcome break from the very tough year I had just finished.

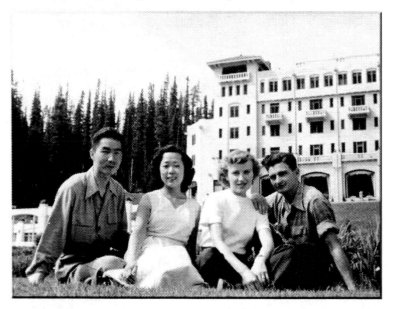

PHOTO 28 [Dr. Ying and wife Winnie, Connie and author]

On arriving back in Vancouver, I immediately began my six-month stint on pediatrics. During this time, since I was not required to do histories on new patients (these were done by the junior interns), I had considerably more time to read and study. I managed to read Nelson's Textbook of Pediatrics from cover to cover - about eighteen hundred pages. I was also able to spend time reading about the various conditions for which our patients had been admitted to hospital. I was also taught a number of procedures which would be of help to me in general practice. For example, I learned the so-called "cutdown" which was used if an infant was going to need intravenous fluids for a number of days. The procedure consisted of making a small incision near the ankle bone. Using a small hook, the vein in this region was grasped and brought to the surface. A small incision was then made into the vein and a polyethylene catheter was threaded into it. An intravenous could then be attached to this tubing when needed.

Also, using a special tiny needle called a butterfly, I learned how to insert it into one of the small veins of the scalp of an infant in order to get a specimen of blood for testing. This could also be used for intravenous feeding. When it was difficult to find a suitable vein in an infant in order to get blood for testing, I learned how to insert a needle deep into the internal jugular vein. With the use of a special needle, and under local anaesthesia, I learned how to get a specimen of bone marrow from the tibia in order to test for anemia or possible leukemia.

One of the most valuable things I learned at this time was how to do a careful and complete examination of the newborn infant. I was taught to look for congenital abnormalities such as club foot, congenital dislocation of the hip, umbilical hernia, possible heart disease, abnormalities of the nasal passages and ear canals. By carefully examining every newborn infant, abnormalities can be spotted quickly and appropriate treatment initiated. I had the opportunity of doing lumbar punctures on infants and young children in order to test the cerebrospinal fluid (CSF) for evidence of infection when meningitis was suspected.

I also had the opportunity to assist in replacement transfusions which were necessary at times in newborn infants born with the condition known as erythroblastosis. This was a severe hemolytic anemia due to the breakdown of the red blood cells caused by the Rh factor when the mother was Rh negative, the father Rh positive and the infant Rh positive. This procedure is not needed nearly so often now because it is possible to prevent erythroblastosis by giving the mother Rh immune globulin at the right time and at the correct dosage. Replacement transfusions were fairly common in 1950.

In 1949, St. Paul's Hospital became the first hospital in British Columbia to develop a nursery for premature infants. At that time, an infant was considered to be premature if it weighed less than five and one-half pounds at birth.

The nursery was designed by Dr. Peter Spohn, who had just returned to Vancouver following a four-year residency in pediatrics at the Johns Hopkins Hospital in Baltimore. I spent as much time as possible in this nursery where I learned to care for these tiny infants who often weighed only two or three pounds. Besides the challenge of feeding these infants, many complications required treatment.

The nurses who worked in this unit had been specially trained to care for these babies. It was amazing to watch them handle these patients with such skill and gentleness. Since I was keen to learn as much as I could concerning the care of these infants, the nurses went out of their way to teach me what they knew. They taught me how to pick up the infants gently so as not to cause them any harm. They showed me how to pass a tiny feeding tube into their stomachs in order to feed them breast milk or specially-prepared formulas. At first, I was hesitant to insert the feeding tube for fear that I might not know whether the tube went down the esophagus and into the stomach, or whether it might have gone into the trachea. The secret was to listen carefully as the feeding tube was threaded down the esophagus. When the tube entered the stomach, a characteristic "pop" could be heard.

These nurses truly loved their work and cared for these infants as if they were their own. They would take them out of the incubators for short periods of time, waltz around the nursery with the infants cradled in their arms, all the while singing softly to them. The smallest infant that was cared for in the nursery weighed a little over one pound. The babies remained in the premature nursery until they weighed five and one-half pounds, at which time they were discharged from hospital.

Some of these infants developed blindness due to a condition called retrolental fibroplasia in which a fibrous substance collected in the fluid (vitreous humor) behind the lens. It would be a number of years before the cause of this condition was identified. While the infants were small, they were kept in incubators with a high concentration of oxygen flowing continually. It was determined that when the oxygen was finally discontinued, the sudden drop in the concentration of oxygen in the incubator resulted in the formation of the fibrous tissue. Once this was recognized and the concentration of oxygen was reduced, the condition no longer developed.

Some of these infants were so premature that they could become blind, deaf or mentally retarded. This created an ethical question as to just how aggressive we should be in caring for such tiny creatures. And so we have reached the situation today where, on the one hand, we have highly-trained doctors and nurses doing everything in their power to save the life of a tiny infant who may have little hope of leading a normal life, while, on the other hand, we have a doctor deliberately taking the life of a potentially normal infant for no other reason than that the mother has decided she does not want the child. He is performing a "therapeutic" abortion. Does this make any sense?

During my time on pediatrics, I learned a good deal about the feeding of infants. This included breast feeding, the use of solid foods, vitamins and special supplements. I learned how to make an accurate diagnosis of a condition called pyloric stenosis. In this condition, a small, benign, muscular tumor forms at the lower end of the stomach causing obstruction at the site of the tumour. During the first few weeks of life, the infant begins to vomit. The vomiting becomes more frequent and more severe as time goes on until the milk actually shoots out of the mouth. This has been labelled "projectile vomiting". By examining the infant carefully with the tips of the fingers of the left hand, the tumor can be felt and rolled beneath the fingers. The tumor feels like a small olive. Once the diagnosis is made correctly, surgical treatment is carried out. The surgery consists of cutting through the muscle fibers down to, but not through, the inner lining of the stomach. This results in a dramatic and permanent cure. My role in the treatment of these babies was to do a cutdown on the morning of the surgery so that intravenous fluids could be administered during the surgery and for a day or two afterwards. I also helped in the post-operative care of these patients.

During my six-month period on the pediatric service, I saw many unusual, and even rare conditions, including an eight-week old infant who developed obstruction of the laryngeal airway from a vascular tumor (hemangioma). A tracheotomy was required in order to relieve the obstruction. After the hemangioma was treated, the otolaryngologist who had performed the tracheotomy removed the tracheotomy tube in the nursery and inserted a smaller tube. This was necessary in order to wean the infant off the tracheotomy tube. He removed the tube without difficulty and inserted a smaller one. However, he did not remain with the infant for a few minutes after changing the tube to be sure everything was all right. About thirty minutes later, a nurse went into the nursery to check on the infant and found him dead. Autopsy revealed that the tracheotomy tube was not in the trachea. It was lying in front of the trachea and over the opening into the windpipe. The infant had died from asphyxia.

In 1950 there were two procedures which were being carried out by some doctors. These procedures were even questionable at that time, but have subsequently been shown not only to be of no use, but to be harmful. At that time (and also presently) there was the occasional case of sudden infant death. For some unknown reason a normal infant would be found dead in his crib. There was no logical explanation for the death. The label "crib death" or "sudden infant death" was applied to these tragic episodes. At autopsy, it was noticed that the thymus gland, which lies behind the upper part of the sternum, was enlarged. At least the gland was thought to be enlarged. It was therefore concluded that the cause of death might be due to pressure of the thymus gland on the underlying trachea causing obstruction of the trachea. The term status-thymico-lymphaticus was coined to explain these sudden deaths. Someone got the idea of treating the thymus gland with radiation, causing it to shrink in size, thereby preventing this mishap. Radiation was applied to the upper chest of these newborn infants before they were discharged from hospital. A number of years were to pass before this so-called prophylactic was discontinued. It became apparent, after hundreds of autopsies on newborn infants, that the thymus gland was normally quite large at birth and gradually decreased in size spontaneously over a period of several months. Statistics also revealed that those infants who had been subjected to this radiation had a much higher incidence of cancer of the thyroid gland when they reached adulthood. This was thought to be due to the radiation.

There was another form of therapy which was popular with some otolaryngologists in the '50s. This consisted of treating the nasopharynx with radium in those children who had persistent regrowth of adenoid tissue after it had been removed surgically. Lymphoid tissue is very sensitive to radiation. Many years later, it was discovered that these children, on reaching adulthood, had a much greater incidence of cancer of the nasopharynx.

The lesson to be learned here is that it behooves the practising physician to retain a certain degree of scepticism for new modes of treatment until it has been proven beyond doubt that they are not only effective, but what is even more important, that they have been shown to cause no harm to the patient.

During my six-month period on the medical service, I was able to review the management of many important conditions. I learned how to manage patients who had been admitted for myocardial infarction with anti-coagulants, how to regulate the diet and insulin requirements of diabetics, how to manage hypertension, peptic ulcer, stroke, pneumonia, congestive heart failure, pulmonary edema, various anemias, allergic conditions and reactions, meningitis, renal disease, diseases of the liver and many, many other conditions. We held arthritis clinics every Wednesday afternoon. At these clinics, I saw dozens of patients with various forms of arthritis, thereby improving my ability not only in making an accurate diagnosis, but also in initiating proper treatment.

As senior intern, it was my responsibility to prepare patients for our weekly teaching rounds in which interesting patients were presented to the hospital medical staff for discussion. I also participated in the presentation of unusual patients at grand rounds, which were carried out every two months.

At the time that I was on the medical service, cortisone was beginning to be used for conditions such as rheumatoid arthritis, various forms of allergy, and some skin conditions. Some people even thought it was the ultimate treatment for erythroblastosis. It was considered to be the Wonder Drug of all. However, time revealed that its uses were limited and that there were many serious complications resulting from the side-effects of the drug, such as osteoporosis, flare-up of latent pulmonary tuberculosis, peptic ulcers with serious bleeding, depression of the adrenal glands, cataracts and a marked gain in weight. Doctors had become too enthusiastic about this Wonder Drug.

Over a period of six months, I saw many patients with interesting and unusual conditions. For example, a man in his middle sixties was brought to the emergency room in a comatose state. He had been found in this condition by his next-door neighbor, who called an ambulance. Examination revealed that he was dehydrated, his eyeballs were sunken, the skin and mucous membranes were dry, his respirations were rapid and deep (so-called Kussmaul breathing), his blood pressure was low and his pulse was rapid and weak. There was an odor of acetone on his breath. He had a large amount of glucose in his urine along with some acetone and the blood sugar was very high. The diagnosis of diabetic coma was made.

An intravenous of isotonic saline was started and plain insulin was added to the I-V bottle. A catheter was inserted into his bladder in order to monitor his output of urine. His pulse, blood pressure, respiration and level of consciousness were checked regularly. He was examined very carefully for any signs of infection, but none was found. The I-V with the insulin was given continuously at a fairly rapid rate. Over a period of several hours he was gradually re-hydrated, his blood sugar returned to normal, the urine became free of glucose and acetone and he gradually regained consciousness.

It was fascinating to observe this patient gradually recover from a comatose state. Within a few days he was discharged from hospital in a healthy state. I was fortunate to have played a part in the treatment of this patient.

In another case, a middle-aged man was admitted to hospital by one of the prominent dermatologists of Vancouver. This patient had a rare condition called generalized exfoliative dermatitis. At the time of admission, his whole body was weeping (raw) except for small areas which were covered with dry, scaly debris.The treatment prescribed by the specialist was to sponge the body with normal saline solution and then to coat it with calamine lotion every six hours using a soft paint brush, in order to reduce the weeping. In spite of treatment, within twenty-four hours of admission to hospital, the patient expired.

Following the discussion of this patient at ward rounds, it was the consensus of opinion that he had died from loss of fluids, protein and electrolytes from the weeping skin. It was felt that he should have been treated vigorously with high-protein intravenous fluids and that his electrolytes should have been monitored carefully and replaced adequately. I was certainly aware that there were very serious dermatological conditions but I was shocked to see a patient die so quickly from one of these.

A boy, six years of age, was admitted to hospital for investigation of persistent headaches. The headaches had begun for no apparent reason and had been present for a number of weeks. The headaches were general in nature, came on shortly after getting out of bed in the morning and subsided as the day went on. However, since their onset, they were occurring more frequently, were more severe and were lasting for longer periods of time. The pain, when it was present, was steady and dull. A day or two prior to admission to hospital, the patient began to experience spells of vomiting which came on for no apparent reason and which were not associated with any nausea.

Physical examination was normal except for one finding. On examining the eyes with an ophthalmoscope, a condition known as papilledema was noted. Papilledema refers to the blurring of the margins of the optic disc. The optic disc is the circular area at the back of the eye where the optic nerve, artery and vein enter the globe. Normally, the margin of the disc is clear and sharp. Blurring of the optic disc is often a sign of increase in the pressure of the cerebrospinal fluid.

X-rays of the skull showed slight widening of the suture (joints) lines due to increase in intracranial pressure of the cerebrospinal fluid. Further investigation revealed a large tumor of the cerebellum. Due to the size and location of the tumor, it was felt that surgical excision was not possible. He was treated with chemotherapy and radiation but had a poor response to this.

Over a period of a few weeks, his condition deteriorated with increasing headache, vomiting, coma and, finally, death. It was sad and frustrating to witness this young boy gradually succumb to this malignancy knowing there was very little that could be done other than to try to keep him free of pain.

One evening, when I was on emergency call, I was asked to see one of the orderlies who was on duty. This fellow was in his mid-forties and had developed sudden, severe abdominal pain. When I saw the patient, he was obviously experiencing severe abdominal pain. He was sitting up on the edge of the bed with his knees drawn up and his hands and forearms folded across the abdomen to exert pressure upon it. He was leaning slightly forward because this position seemed to lessen the pain somewhat.

The pain was located in the centre of the upper abdomen (epigastrium), was steady, boring in nature and radiated into the back. I asked him to lie down on his back, and although this increased the pain, he was very co-operative while I carried out my examination. He was obviously in great distress, anxious and restless. His skin was cold and sweaty. His pulse was rapid and his blood pressure was below what would be expected for his age indicating a degree of shock. The whole abdomen was tender, but more so in the epigastrium. The muscles of the abdomen were tense, but not board-like as seen with a perforated peptic ulcer. There were no bowel sounds audible.

Although I had never seen a patient with this condition before, I felt that the most likely diagnosis was acute pancreatitis. I phoned Dr. Hurlburt and asked him to see the patient. Dr. Hurlburt was the most competent internist I have ever known, possibly with the exception of Dr. John Scott, head of the

Department of Medicine at the University of Alberta at that time. After seeing the patient, ordering a number of lab tests and abdominal x-rays, Dr. Hurlburt confirmed the diagnosis of acute pancreatitis. With vigorous medical treatment, the patient recovered completely.

Acute pancreatitis is an inflammation of the pancreas, an exocrine and endocrine gland situated in the upper abdomen. The exocrine portion of the gland produces pancreatic juice, which contains various enzymes that are important in the digestion of foods. The endocrine portion consists of the Islets of Langerhans, which produce insulin and other hormones. Acute pancreatitis is most often associated with alcoholism or disease of the biliary tract. During the disease process, the enzymes digest the pancreatic tissue and blood vessels. The severity of the process can vary considerably and the mortality rate can vary from five percent to eighty percent depending upon the severity of the condition.

Although we worked very hard during our two years of internship, it was not all work and no play. The hospital paid for annual memberships to the YMCA for the interns. Since the "Y" was only one block from the hospital, we would often run down there during visiting hours to play handball or go for a swim. When we were not busy, we would play cards and other games in the small lounge situated in the living quarters of the interns. One of the favorite games was four-handed solitaire in which each player used a deck of cards. Sometimes there was utter bedlam during these games.

On Saturday nights, those who were not on duty would occasionally rent the arena at Hasting's Park in order to play hockey for a couple of hours. We stopped doing this after Pat Doyle ran into the boards one night and fractured his wrist.

One Saturday night, a group of us went to the Cave Night Club and danced to the music of Louis Armstrong. That was a night to remember. Another time, we went to one of the other clubs downtown to listen to and dance to the Ink Spots.

One of the interns liked to party on Saturday nights. On one occasion, when he came back to the interns' quarters quite inebriated, we undressed him, held him under a cold shower for several minutes and then pushed him out into the hallway. He stood there naked and shouting and pounding on the glass door until one of the nursing sisters spotted him while she was on the way to the pharmacy. We let him sweat it out for a couple of minutes longer and then opened the door to let him back into the quarters.

Another night, when this same intern came back to the quarters after a night on the town we carried him up to the plaster room and put a plaster cast on him. We then carried him back to his room and dumped him into his bed. When he awakened in the morning and found himself immobilized in the cast, he began to holler. We finally got him to quiet down so that one of us could remove the cast with the

Stryker Saw. However, these two lessons were still not enough to deter his excessive drinking on Saturday nights

Another intern who appeared a bit different than the others had come from Dublin, Ireland. At that time, every graduate of a foreign medical school was required to spend one year in an approved hospital before being eligible to take the Canadian examinations. He had arranged to take this year at St. Paul's.

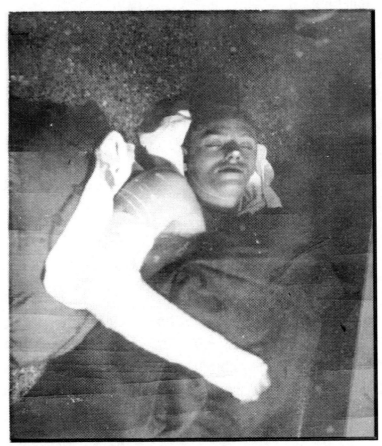

PHOTO 29 [Photo of partying intern in a cast]

In our day it was the custom for interns (and practising physicians) to carry their stethoscopes in their pockets when they were not being used. What made the Irish intern different from the rest of us was that he draped his stethoscope around his neck when he was not using it. Everyone kidded him about this. After a few weeks of teasing, he kept his stethoscope in his pocket like the rest of us.

What reminded me of this rather insignificant event is that over the past year or two I have noticed that anyone who is remotely involved in health care has a stethoscope. Where do you suppose they keep this instrument when it is not in use – draped around their necks!

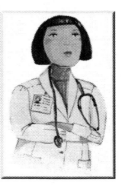

PHOTO 30 [Photo of person with stethoscope around neck]

Whenever doctors or nurses appear on television, there is this ever-present stethoscope. I couldn't help shaking my head one evening as I watched the CBC News. A doctor who had been doing genetic research for many years was being interviewed about her work. Although she probably hadn't used a stethoscope since she interned many years ago, what do you think was dangling from her neck? You guessed it. Not only have members of the medical and nursing professions adopted this silly habit, but chiropractors, veterinarians and anyone who is involved in the health of humans or animals is doing it. It has become the *sine qua non* of the caregiver.

I will always have fond memories of the two years I spent at St. Paul's. I began those two years as a young medical graduate with some theoretical knowledge of medicine, surgery and obstetrics and completed them with considerable practical experience. However, I was soon to learn that competency in the practice of medicine requires never-ending study which must continue for as long as one remains in active practice.

CHAPTER 8: THE JOURNEY TO
THE CARIBOO

Am I Ready For The Real World?

The cure of the disease must never be worse than the disease itself.
Avicenna, Arabian Physician

On June 4, 1951, after a twenty-hour labor, my wife Connie delivered our first son, Phil. A couple of weeks later, Connie flew back to Edmonton with Phil to visit her parents. While she was in Edmonton, I met Dr. Frank Avery, who had driven down from Quesnel to Vancouver to try to find a doctor who might be interested in giving him a hand. I spoke with Dr. Avery in the coffee shop of the hospital and decided that I would like to go to Quesnel for a year or two to get some experience. I phoned Connie to explain things to her and to ask what she thought about it. The first question she asked was *"Where is Quesnel?"*. I had also asked this question because I must admit that I had never heard of the Village of Quesnel. In any event, Connie agreed to give it a try.

Dr. Avery was the only doctor working full time in Quesnel at that time. Dr. Gerald Baker was semi-retired and went to the office for a couple of hours twice a week. Dr. Jarv Tompkins had been in Quesnel for a year but had just recently left Quesnel to join his brother, who was a doctor in Vulcan, Alberta.

In the early morning of July 15, 1951, we left Vancouver on our long drive to Quesnel. The present freeway was non-existent and so we departed from Vancouver by travelling along Kingsway Avenue to New Westminster. After crossing the Pattullo Bridge, we travelled along the Fraser Highway, passing through towns such as Whalley, Surrey, Langley, Clearbrook and Abbotsford until we reached the town of Hope. It took us over three hours to reach Hope from Vancouver. After stopping for a bite to eat, we turned north and headed for the historical Cariboo Highway. A few miles north of Hope, we passed through Yale and began our exciting journey over the Cariboo road.

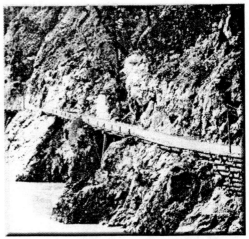

PHOTO 31 [The Cariboo Highway in 1951]

This road was nothing like it is today. The highway was narrow, very winding and followed the Fraser Canyon closely. There were places where only one car could pass at a time. If another car was coming from the opposite direction, the car on the inside of the road would have to back up until a place was reached which was wide enough to allow two cars to pass. There were some places where it had not been possible to carve a road out of the rocky cliffs. In these places, trestles were constructed outward from the cliffs so that the road was literally hanging from the cliff over the Fraser River. The tunnels that had been cut through the mountains were very narrow and pitch black. As we entered these tunnels, we felt that there would not be enough room for two cars to pass.

We continued along the highway to Boston Bar, a tiny railroad town. Just north of Boston Bar, we spotted a small creek on the right side of the road.

We stopped, got out of the car and found a few fellow travellers who were sitting in the shade by the creek.

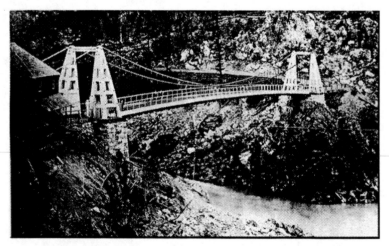

PHOTO 32 [Old Alexandra Bridge in 1951]

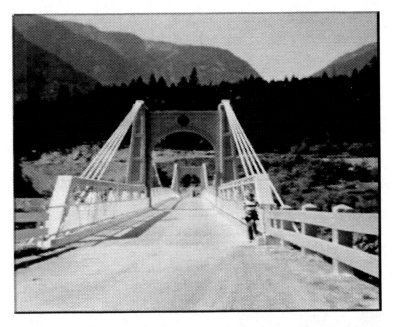

PHOTO 33 [Author's wife standing at the entrance to Alexandra Bridge]

It was like an oasis in the desert. After a short rest, we continued along the Cariboo Highway until we reached the Village of Lytton. I stopped the car at the top of a hill and we got out to stretch our legs. We had a beautiful view of the canyon below us where the blue Thompson River emptied into the muddy Fraser River.

After a brief rest, we continued our journey to Spences Bridge where we stopped for sandwiches and a cool drink. It took over three hours to cover the twisty road from Yale to Spences Bridge. After lunch, we continued north to Cache Creek where the highway divided, one road leading east to Kamloops

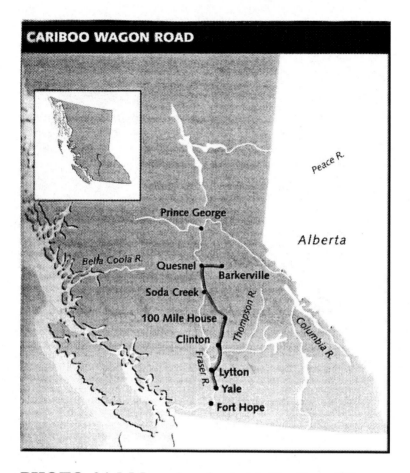

PHOTO 34 [Map showing old Cariboo Wagon Road]

and the other continuing north. We carried on along the north road until we reached the 150 Mile House where I suddenly found myself driving on a hard, rocky road. After going a short distance, I turned around and headed back to the blacktop. I thought that I had somehow driven off the highway and onto a side road. I drove up to the autowrecker at the top of the hill (still there by the way) and asked the owner where the highway was. He remarked *"You've just come off it"*. So we headed back to the heavily gravelled highway and carried on to Williams Lake.

From Williams Lake we followed the Fraser River, up and down hills, around curves and over wooden bridges until we landed in Quesnel four hours later. It had taken four hours to drive the seventy-five miles from Williams Lake to Quesnel. We arrived in Quesnel just before dark and decided to spend the night in the first motel we saw, which was Trites Auto Court. I phoned Dr. Avery to let him know that we had arrived and to find out where we were going to be living for the next couple of years.

The next morning Dr. Avery drove us to a little house on Front Street, half a block from the office and the hospital. That afternoon, the moving van with our furniture arrived from Vancouver, but the driver refused to unload it until I had paid him the four hundred dollars moving charges. I had to borrow the money from Dr. Avery.

The house was small but comfortable. There was a kitchen, living room, bathroom and two bedrooms. There was no such thing as central heating with a furnace. The whole house was heated by the kitchen stove, which was a sawdust burner. Connie had never seen a sawdust burner, but it didn't take her long to get used to it. The first thing I did was to buy a fridge, which I managed to get second-hand from Bruce Stanbridge for one hundred dollars.

It didn't take us long to settle in. I was busy from the first day I started practising and would remain so until I left Quesnel two years later.

In 1951, Quesnel was a Village of about one thousand people. It also served a large surrounding area extending north to Hixon, south to Marguerite, west to the Nazko Valley and east to Barkerville and Wells. There were roughly about another thousand people in this surrounding area. The only industry in Quesnel was logging. There were about two hundred small sawmills in the area, but the major single employer was the Western Plywood Plant. Most of the roads in the Village were gravel. There was a single paved road (a combination of Front Street and Carson Avenue) which were, and still are, part of Highway No. 97.

The telephones were the old-fashioned type which required cranking. Our call number was one long and three short. To call someone, we lifted the receiver, and when the operator answered, we asked her to get us that particular person. There was only one telephone outside of the Village and that was at the store immediately across the bridge over the Fraser River, in West Quesnel. At midnight, when the switchboard operator went off duty, she would connect the telephones of the hospital, the RCMP office and the doctor on call. No other phones in the Village were operative after midnight. The only way a patient could get a doctor would be to go to the doctor's home or to the hospital and ask the nurse to call him.

As a matter of interest, in the early sixties, the B.C. Telephone Company modernized the system in Quesnel. Alex Fraser, our former next-door neighbour, was the Mayor of Quesnel at the time. The day that the switch was thrown to bring the new system into operation, Alex was allowed to place the first call to any place he chose in North America. Connie and I were surprised and delighted when he decided to phone us in Richmond, Virginia, where I was doing post-graduate work at the time.

The Quesnel Clinic was located in a tiny bungalow across from the hospital on Front Street. There was a small waiting room which would seat about eight people, a room for the receptionist and bookkeeper, a tiny room in the centre of the building with a sink and sterilizer, a small emergency room and two small examining rooms for the doctors.

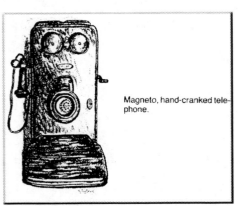

Magneto, hand-cranked telephone.

PHOTO 35 [Diagram of type of telephone in use in Quesnel in the early 1950s]

There was no hot water tap nor laboratory facilities. The building was heated by means of a wood furnace which was located in a tiny basement. Dr. Avery and I were the only doctors working full time. Dr. Baker, who had been in Quesnel for many years, came to the office two afternoons a week in order to see patients whom he had cared for for many years.

The hospital was a wooden, two storey, frame building. There was a small office for the hospital administrator, Bill Speare, and a large ward on the first floor for male patients. This would hold about eight patients. There was a tiny room which we used for children. There was a small operating room and a tiny x-ray room. The only person who knew how to operate the x-ray machine was Flora Tingley, the matron. She was able to take pictures of the skull, chest, arms and legs, and that was it.

The second floor of the hospital consisted of one large room for female patients, two small rooms for patients, a tiny labor room and a delivery room.

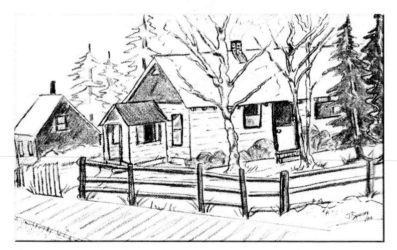

PHOTO 36 [Diagram of the Quesnel Medical Clinic on Front Street, Quesnel – Drawn by Mrs. Jean Speare]

There was no running hot water available in the hospital so that when we scrubbed for surgery, we used green soap and cold water. Since there was no elevator in the building, it was necessary to carry female patients from the operating room, up the stairs, to the second floor. In order to get around the corner while going up the stairs, it was necessary to tilt the head of the stretcher downward.

The only anaesthetics used at that time were local novocain or xylocaine, nerve blocks, spinals

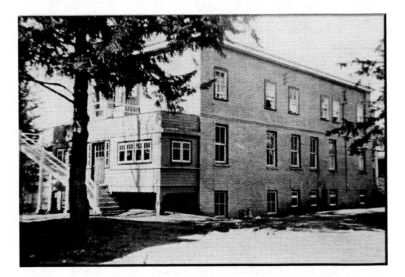

PHOTO 37 [The Quesnel Hospital in 1951]

with heavy pontocaine, pentothal for short anaesthesia requiring no relaxation, and open-drop ether for general anaesthesia. We started the general anaesthetic using an ether mask and Vinethene (Vinyl ether), which is a very quick-acting ether. Within about thirty seconds the patient would be asleep.

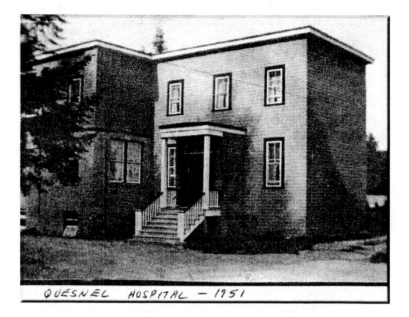

QUESNEL HOSPITAL — 1951

PHOTO 38 [Hospital on Front Street in 1951]

We would then switch over to open-drop ether and pour this from an ether can with a cork partially obstructing it so that we could control the rate of flow. It would take several minutes to get the patient anaesthetized deeply enough before the surgery could be started.

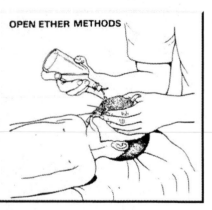

OPEN ETHER METHODS

PHOTO 39 [Drawing of open-drop ether method used in 1951-52]

Spinal anaesthetics were used for surgery of the legs, pelvis and lower abdomen. Most fractures did not require a long anaesthetic, unless we had to do an open reduction and plating, so we used pentothal for these procedures. An open reduction refers to the procedure of making an incision over the fracture site, exposing the ends of the broken bones and manipulating them into proper alignment. A stainless steel plate is then placed over the fracture site and held in place with four or more stainless steel screws. The incision is then closed with sutures and a plaster cast applied in order to prevent the bones from moving out of alignment.

In 1951, the administrator of the hospital was Bill Speare. He was always supportive of any suggestions the members of the medical staff made which might improve the quality of care. Bill had been a tank commander during WWII. He had been wounded which resulted in the loss of his right arm just below the shoulder joint. Prior to his enlistment in the army, he had been an artist. The loss of his right arm must have been a terrible blow to him. However, he was the type of person who was able to recover from adversity and taught himself to paint with his left hand.

While I was in Quesnel, Bill resigned his position as administrator in order to enter politics. He was subsequently elected as the M.L.A. for the Cariboo. For reasons unknown to me, he resigned after a very short period of time.

As a matter of interest, in 1965, after doing post-graduate work in the United States, I was invited to speak to the doctors in Williams Lake. At that time, I had the opportunity of renewing acquaintances with Bill who was doing an excellent job as administrator of the Cariboo Memorial Hospital in Williams Lake.

Prior to my journey to Quesnel, I had spent two years working in the largest city in British Columbia, in a modern hospital, with all of the up-to-date equipment available at that time. Now I was embarking on a country practice in a remote Village with no modern facilities nor equipment. The treatment of my patients would be determined entirely upon my ability to take a good history and to follow this with a very careful physical examination. I was going to need a lot of help from the power above.

In spite of this shocking introduction to family practice, I was not the least bit fearful of accepting the challenge. You might call it the folly of youth. Perhaps it was the magnitude of the challenge which appealed to me. At any rate, I was never sorry for having made the decision to go to the Cariboo country.

When I look back now and compare the situation which existed even in the major centres at that time, with what is available now, we had not really come that far in the practice of medicine, surgery and obstetrics compared to what is available in 2005.

CHAPTER 9 – INTRODUCTION TO COUNTRY PRACTICE

The Action Begins

There are few occupations of a more satisfying character than the practice of medicine.
Sir William Osler

In 1951, when I arrived in Quesnel, the medical personnel and hospital situation in the Cariboo region consisted of the following: as mentioned already, in Quesnel, there was a two-storey, wooden-framed hospital. There were two doctors, Dr. Frank Avery and Dr. Gerald Baker. In Prince George, there was a single-storey, wooden-framed hospital, shaped like the spokes of a wheel and converted from an army barracks. There were seven doctors, all of them general practitioners. In Williams Lake, there was a two-storey, wooden-framed hospital. There was one doctor, Larry Avery.

In Wells, there was a two-storey building. There was one doctor, Dr. Berera. At 100 Mile House, there was no hospital and no doctor. At Lytton, there was a single-storey, wooden-framed hospital. There was one doctor. At Ashcroft, there was a single-storey, wooden-framed hospital. There was one doctor. At that time, there were no specialists north of Kamloops in the Province of British Columbia, with the exception of Alf Mooney, who was a certified general surgeon practising in Vanderhoof.

We arrived in Quesnel on a Saturday evening and I started to see patients on Monday morning. The following weekend, Dr. Avery left town to visit his brother Larry who was the only doctor in Williams Lake at the time. I didn't mind Dr. Avery going out of town since he hadn't had a break in several weeks. He deserved a rest. I was very busy all weekend seeing emergencies at the hospital.

Besides seeing patients with the usual cuts, bruises, sprains and sore throats, two patients in particular remain in my memory. One was a young man who, while repairing the roof of his house, lost his footing and fell about twenty feet to the ground. He was brought to the hospital and found to have a fracture of the neck of the right femur. Since this would require an open reduction and nailing, I phoned Dr. McConkey in Vancouver and arranged to send the patient down to St. Paul's Hospital on the next plane. In the meantime, I immobilized the leg in a Thomas splint and kept him comfortable with morphine.

The other patient was a middle-aged man who had taken a fall while coming down the back stairs of his house, resulting in a fracture of the lower end of the right radius (so-called Colles fracture). Since I had no one to give an anaesthetic, I decided to inject the fracture site with Novocain. We reduced the fracture by my grasping his hand and thumb and exerting traction, while he pulled against me. We had no problem in reducing the fracture in this manner after which I applied a plaster cast in order to immobilize the arm until healing had occurred.

Although I had been a bit apprehensive about being the only doctor in town after my first week of practice, fortunately there were no serious emergencies requiring the expertise of two or more doctors. However, I must admit that I breathed a sigh of relief when Sunday evening arrived and Dr. Avery returned.

When I reflect and compare Quesnel to similar small towns in B.C. at the present time, I am amazed at the changes which have occurred. Besides the limited office and hospital facilities which we had in 1951, there was no such thing as medicare and there were no specialists nearby whom we could call upon if we needed expert help. Due to the long distance and time required to travel from Quesnel to Kamloops, it was easier and quicker to refer patients with the more serious injuries and illnesses to Vancouver and to have them travel by plane.

At that time, there was no such thing as air-ambulance service in the interior of B.C. The planes patients travelled on to get to Vancouver were the regular CPA flights which travelled from Prince George to Vancouver with a ten-minute stop-over at Quesnel once a day. If weather was not good and the visibility was poor, the plane did not stop in Quesnel.

One of the early surgical procedures I was called upon to do was a hemorrhoidectomy. I had assisted at a number of these operations and had witnessed others carried out by Dr. Whaley, who had been dubbed "the Rear Admiral" by one of the interns. Dr. Whaley had restricted his surgery to doing hemorrhoidectomies and nothing else – talk about specialization! He was way ahead of his time. However, I was a little leery of doing my first real surgical procedure alone so I asked Dr. Baker if he would mind assisting me.

One Sunday, I was relaxing at home when there was a knock on the door. When I opened it, Dr. Baker was standing there with a box in his hand. I invited him in and asked him what he was carrying. He produced a cigar box, which he opened. Inside were dozens of pieces of ribbons of different colors, various feathers, threads and hooks. He said that he wanted to leave these with me and that he would be back one day to give me some lessons on tying flies. He felt that as long as I was living in the Cariboo, I would have to learn how to fish and to hunt.

A couple of days before our first Christmas in Quesnel, Dr. Baker appeared at our front door again. This time he was carrying a Winchester shotgun. He said that he and Mrs. Baker wanted to give the gun to me as a Christmas present. The gun had been owned by Mrs. Baker's father. She must have thought quite a bit of me to give me such a gift.

The only time I ever used the gun was the day Dr. Baker and I drove along the Six-Mile Road. He had picked me up in his truck and was going to give me my first hunting lesson. Half-way up the hill, Dr. Baker stopped his truck and we got out. We strolled into the bush and before long a bird flew out in front of us. I aimed the gun quickly and pulled the trigger.

By some miracle, I hit the bird. Dr. Baker picked it up and walked back to me. It was an owl!

He complimented me and said he would take the bird and give it to the Chinese cook at the Nugget Restaurant. According to Dr. Baker, the cook loved owl's meat. It was his favourite. I was a little dubious, but took his word for it. I'll never know if he was telling me the truth or just trying to make me feel good.

Dr. Baker used to invite me over to his house occasionally for a visit. Mrs. Baker would pour me a small glass of sherry and give me a couple of cookies. I never enjoyed the taste of sherry, but I always drank it with a look of pleasure as I didn't want her to think that I did not appreciate her thoughtfulness. The two of them were always very kind to me.

I had a large medical bag which had been given to me as a graduation present by our family doctor. This bag was my companion on every house call that I ever made. It held the usual diagnostic instruments such as stethoscope, otoscope, ophthalmoscope, sphygmomanometer (for checking blood pressure), reflex hammer, oral and rectal thermometers (a little different in shape to prevent any error in use), sterile latex gloves and sterile urethral catheter. There was a special syringe and ampoules of penicillin, ampoules of adrenalin and other odds and ends. Remember that a house call might take me several miles out of town into the bush or a logging camp. In view of this, it would not be a simple matter of giving a patient a prescription to be filled at the corner pharmacy.

I had a special spotlight attached to the front of my car that I could direct by means of a handle located handily inside the car near the steering wheel. This was very helpful to me at times when I was trying to locate a house in pitch-black darkness, or when I was on a strange road and might risk getting stuck if the wheels strayed from the packed mud or snow.

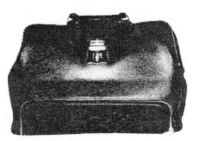

PHOTO 40 [Photo of medical bag which was a graduation present – carried essential equipment on house calls]

I always carried a tow-chain in the trunk of my car. This was needed on a number of occasions when I had gotten stuck in thick mud or had slid off the packed portion of the road in winter and sank down into deep snow. At such times, I would wait for a logging truck to come along and would use the tow-chain in order to help the trucker pull my car back onto the road.

I always had two complete sets of wheels for my car. One set was mounted with ordinary summer tires, while the other set was mounted with winter tires all of which were studded.

During the early 1950s, although most of the roads were named, none of the houses had numbers.

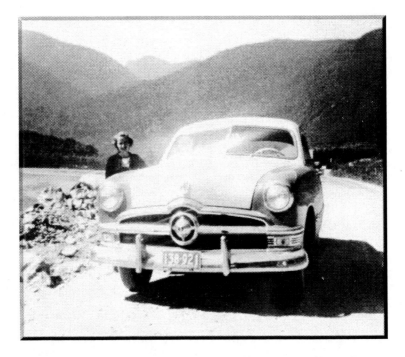

PHOTO 41 [Photo of author's wife Connie, standing by 1950 Ford used for hundreds of house calls]

It was not unusual to be given directions such as "I live two houses past John Smith in a log cabin" or " I'm half a mile past the community hall on the right side of the road in a white cottage" or "Do you know where Bob Brown lives? I'll meet you in front of his house and drive the rest of the way with you". It didn't take many months before I knew where most people lived as well as every landmark in Quesnel and for miles around.

I believe the thing I enjoyed the most about doing general practice in the Cariboo was the great variety of conditions I was required to treat. I never knew what I might be faced with next. A doctor who has never done this type of work has missed one of the real joys of practising medicine.

During my time in Quesnel, I made hundreds of house calls, some of them as far as twenty or thirty miles out of town. Many of these calls were to deal with ordinary illnesses, but there was the occasional unusual incident.

On one occasion, the nurse on duty at the hospital phoned me to say that they had received a call for help from someone on the highway, about twenty miles south of town. There was no mention of what the problem was. I grabbed my bag, jumped into the car and headed down the highway.

When I neared Kersley, I noticed a car parked on the side of the road. There were several people standing beside it. I pulled up and got out. I was approached by a man in his thirties, his wife and two children. He told me that they were on their way home to Seattle from Alaska. His mother, who was travelling with them, had developed sudden chest pain and, within a few seconds, had died. She was in the back seat of his car.

I suggested that we transfer the mother to my car and that I take her back to the funeral parlor in Quesnel. They could follow me into town, have dinner at one of the restaurants and afterwards contact the funeral director in order to make the necessary arrangements to have the body transported to Seattle for burial. We transferred the body to my car and I headed into town.

I drove to the funeral parlor of John Harvey, but there was no one there. I drove over to John's home but was informed by Mrs. Harvey that her husband was attending a meeting of the Lion's Club. It was starting to get dark. I went over to the restaurant where the Lion's Club was holding its monthly meeting and found John having dinner. I advised him of what had happened and that I would like to get rid of the passenger who was occupying the back seat of my car.

We drove over to the funeral parlor, transferred the body to John's care, after which I headed for home for a late dinner. As I was driving home, I began to wonder what people might have thought if they had discovered a corpse lying on the back seat of my car.

On another occasion, I was asked to make a house call to the Moffat ranch, which was located a few miles south of town. A young woman who was visiting the Moffats and who was pregnant, had suddenly started to have strong labor pains. The Moffats did not want to take the risk of driving into town for fear that the woman might have the baby during the journey.

When I arrived at the ranch house, I was shown into the kitchen. Sitting in the kitchen were three women. When they saw me, they pointed to the direction of the stove. The oven door of the stove was open, there was a basket lying on the open door and inside of the basket was a tiny baby. After checking the infant and the mother to be sure they were all right, I took them back to the hospital with me.

A young woman who had recently moved from Prince George to Quesnel came in to see me for prenatal care for her third pregnancy. The two previous pregnancies had been uneventful except that the second infant developed jaundice within twenty-four hours of birth. The jaundice had cleared spontaneously with no apparent ill effects. The history was suggestive of mild hemolytic disease of the newborn (erythroblastosis). This became more suspicious when I learned later that my patient's blood type was O Rh-negative.

The pregnancy and delivery of this woman were unremarkable except that the infant was slightly jaundiced at birth. At the time of delivery, I obtained a sample of umbilical cord blood in order to have it tested. Since we had no laboratory facilities in Quesnel at the time, I drove to the hospital in Prince George in order to have the blood checked.

The infant was found to be moderately anemic, the bilirubin level was elevated, the blood type was Rh-positive and the Coombs test was positive. The Coombs test is a special test used to detect antibodies which are attached to the red blood cells and the positive result confirmed the diagnosis. The infant had hemolytic disease and would require replacement transfusion. I obtained a pint of fresh blood, type O, Rh-negative from the hospital and headed back to Quesnel.

Soon after arriving in Quesnel, with the help of Dr. Appleby, we did a replacement transfusion on the newborn infant. We threaded a catheter into the umbilical vein, and with the use of a special syringe, we aspirated 20 millilitres of blood from the infant and infused 20 millilitres of the fresh O-negative blood. We repeated the procedure over and over again until we had infused the whole 500 millilitres of blood. It took about two hours to complete the transfusion. This procedure was considered effectual in replacing ninety percent of the infant's blood.

Erythroblastosis (also known as hemolytic disease of the newborn) is caused by an incompatibility between fetal and maternal blood. The Rh-negative mother becomes immunized by exposure to Rh-positive erythrocytes during pregnancy or delivery, and antibodies formed by the mother pass through the placenta to the fetal circulation where they react with the Rh-positive fetal erythrocytes causing them to break down (hemolytic anemia).

Advances in therapy have dramatically reduced perinatal mortality. Rh-immune globulin is now available and can prevent the condition if given to the mother at the appropriate time and in the correct dosage. If the fetus is known to have hemolytic anemia, intrauterine transfusions can be given to the infant before delivery by injecting blood into the fetal peritoneal cavity or into the fetal umbilical vein. In spite of improved therapy, hemolytic disease of the newborn continues to be an important cause of anemia and jaundice in newborn infants. If the condition is not recognized and treated properly while the infant is still in the uterus, replacement transfusion may still be necessary.

In this particular case, the baby had no problem during the transfusion, the jaundice cleared completely over a few days and, so far as I am aware, there have been no complications.

One afternoon I had a middle-aged man come into my office in a bit of a panic. He was a scrap-iron dealer and travelled regularly from Vancouver to Prince George. He would load his truck with scrap iron and take the truckload back to Vancouver.

He had been to Prince George the previous week, had returned to Vancouver to dump his load and was now on his way back to Prince George to get another load of scrap iron. He had just stopped in Quesnel to gas up, had gone to the washroom to urinate and was shocked when he noticed a purulent discharge coming from the opening of the urethra. He paid the gas attendant quickly and made a beeline for our office.

When I examined him, he had a thick, creamy discharge which could be expressed from the urethra. After taking a smear of the discharge in order to have the diagnosis confirmed, he was given 100,000 units of penicillin intramuscularly. This was the recommended treatment for acute gonorrhea at that time.

I attempted to get the name and address of his contact so that she might be contacted by the Public Health Department and treated. However, he had no idea who had transmitted the infection to him. He told me that whenever he made a trip to Prince George, after he had completed his business, he spent the evening drinking and consorting with prostitutes.

I gave him the usual warning about the high probability of picking up infection with this type of behaviour and sent him on his way.

Approximately a month later, this fellow showed up at my office again. I said jokingly to him *"I guess you didn't learn your lesson the last time you visited Prince George"*. He laughed and replied *"I'm on my way to Prince George right now and I'd like you to give me a shot of penicillin so I won't have to worry while I'm having a good time"*. Of course I had to tell him that penicillin was used only for the treatment of gonorrhea and not as a prophylaxis.

One day a married woman in her mid-twenties was seen in the office because she had awakened that morning with blurring of the vision of her right eye. Examination of that eye with the ophthalmoscope revealed the optic disc to be abnormal. The other eye was normal. The patient had no other symptoms. A complete physical examination was normal.

I referred the patient to Dr. John Ragan, an ophthalmologist and classmate of mine practising in Vancouver. John wrote me a letter after seeing this young lady and advised me that she had a condition called optic neuritis. This condition could be caused by a number of things, the most common being multiple sclerosis. In a high percentage of patients, the first sign of multiple sclerosis is blurring of vision caused by optic neuritis. As it turned out, within a few months, this patient went on to develop other signs and symptoms of multiple sclerosis.

The husband of one of my maternity patients was seen in the office with a pretty embarrassing problem for him. He had awakened that morning with a very itchy and sore penis. When I examined him, the penis was swollen and the skin exhibited a red, blotchy eruption. On questioning him carefully I learned that the previous evening, prior to having intercourse, his wife had used a new spermicidal jelly on her diaphragm. He had been very sensitive to chemicals in the jelly and had developed a severe case of contact dermatitis. He was quite relieved to learn the cause of his problems. This responded quickly to treatment.

One of the old-time ranchers of the Cariboo appeared in my office because he had noticed swelling of his right arm a few days prior to my seeing him. When I examined him, the right arm was swollen from the shoulder to the wrist. The veins over the right side of his chest were very prominent and the lymph nodes of the axilla (armpit) were enlarged and firm. A chest X-ray revealed an area of consolidation in his right lung.

I felt that he might have bronchogenic carcinoma (cancer) of the right lung with metastases (spread) to the lymph nodes. He was referred to a thoracic surgeon who did a bronchoscopy and biopsy which confirmed the diagnosis of lung cancer. He lived for only a few months after having surgery.

I was called to the hospital one evening to see a young girl of about five years of age who had been brought into the emergency room by her mother. This little girl had managed to get into a bottle of pills which her mother had been taking in order to help her lose weight. Fortunately, the mother knew exactly how many pills had remained in the bottle so she was able to determine that her daughter had swallowed only two of them. As a precaution, I felt that we should admit the child to the hospital in order to observe her for a few hours.

These pills belonged to the group of stimulants known as amphetamines. It wasn't long before their stimulating effect began to show itself. The girl began to behave as though she had drunk a couple of cups of coffee. She chattered continually. She never stopped moving for a second. She climbed in and out of her bed. She wandered all over the ward and out into the hallway. This incessant activity went on all night.

She reminded me of one of those old silent movies where the actors were constantly on the move at about three times the normal speed. After a period of a few hours, the effects of the stimulant began to wear off and she enjoyed a long period of sleep.

One of the first babies that I delivered in Quesnel had a mild type of club foot called metatarsus varus. Unless the doctor looks specifically for this condition it can, and often is, missed. I had never really seen this condition when I was in medical school, nor during my hospital training, so I really wasn't sure whether or not it required treatment. With this condition, the inner margin of the foot, instead of being straight, is curved so that the foot has the so-called pigeon-toed shape. As I was unaware of what to do for this, I arranged to have the infant seen by Dr. McConkey. He advised me that treatment was definitely indicated, and that the sooner it was initiated the better the result. He placed the baby's feet in what are known as Dennis-Browne boots. These were tiny leather boots which were worn constantly by the baby. The soles of the boots were attached to a metal bar and the feet were rotated outward ninety degrees. These boots were worn constantly for six weeks. When the boots were removed, the feet were absolutely straight and remained that way.

I obtained a couple of sets of Dennis-Browne boots from the Children's Hospital and over a period of a number of years treated several infants who were born with this condition. The results were always good. If metatarsus varus is not recognized at birth and treated early, the results are not nearly as good. The child might be mildly pigeon-toed permanently.

While I was in Quesnel, I saw only one case of syphilis, but I saw a number of cases of gonorrhea. One patient was a teen-aged son of one of our more prominent citizens. He contracted the infection when he was out of town for a few days. Another was the husband of one of my maternity patients. He went astray after having too much to drink. He was quite embarrassed and guilt-ridden for his behaviour.

On many occasions I had to remind myself of a warning that was given to us in medical school by the professor of obstetrics. He emphasized the warning by telling us a little story. *"A woman comes in to see you with a delicate problem she is having. At that time, she is the only one who is aware of this problem"*. The professor then makes a **1** on the blackboard with a piece of chalk. *"The woman then relates her problem to you, her doctor"*. He makes a second mark on the blackboard beside the first – **11**. *"Now how many people know of the woman's problem?"* All of us, of course, say *"two"*. *"That evening you go home and you tell your wife of this woman's problem"*. He makes a third mark on the blackboard beside the other two – **111**. *"Now, how many people know of this patient's problem?"* The students all say *"three"*.

"Wrong", says the professor. *"Now one hundred and eleven people will know of this woman's*

problem. Your spouse will not be able to contain herself until she relates this woman's problem to the members of her weekly bridge gathering. Never discuss patients' problems with your spouse."

There are so many individuals who come in contact, one way or another, with patients and their records, that it is impossible to retain anything resembling confidentiality; members of the family, friends, the family doctor, his nurse and receptionist, specialists who have seen the patient on referral plus his office staff, laboratory technicians, x-ray technicians, hospital nurses, nursing students, medical students, pharmacists and many others, such as government employees and insurance companies. Today confidentiality does not seem to be nearly as important as it was years ago. However, there does not appear to be any suitable solution to this dilemma.

In the ten years that I was in practice in Quesnel, I had **ONE** patient who requested an abortion. Unbelievable, you might say, but nevertheless, it is true. The patient was in her mid-thirties and lived about twenty miles south of Quesnel, on the west side of the Fraser River.

She told me the following story. Her husband was a logger, which necessitated his being away from home for periods of two or three weeks at a time. While her husband was away, a neighour of hers was kind enough to help her with various chores such as cutting and piling wood, shovelling snow from the driveway and minor repairs to the house.

One day, after he had brought in some firewood, she remarked how generous and helpful he had been. She asked him if there wasn't something she could do for him in return for his generosity. She was taken aback when he replied that he would appreciate it very much if she would allow him to sleep with her (he was a bachelor). After recovering from her surprise, she invited him into her bed.

As luck would have it, she became pregnant. Besides not wanting to have any more children, how would she explain the pregnancy to her husband? She decided that the only solution would be for her to have an abortion. After examining her, I confirmed that she was indeed pregnant as she suspected. I had to explain to her that abortion was illegal under the Criminal Code of Canada and that I would lose my license if I was convicted of performing an abortion. She left my office, somewhat saddened, and I never saw her again.

When you compare this situation with the present condition in Canada insofar as abortion is concerned, it's almost unbelievable that things could have changed so rapidly. Since the Criminal Code was amended in 1969, and abortion was decriminalized, there have been thousands of abortions performed.

At the present time, there are over one hundred thousand abortions performed every year in Canada. Since there is no medical reason for performing these abortions, the majority of fetuses are normal. The sad thing, to my way of thinking, is that there are thousands of women who are unable to conceive, for various reasons, and who would give anything to be able to adopt these babies. The truth of the matter is that there are few babies available for adoption any more. If they are not wanted by the mother, they are aborted. What a waste of potentially healthy Canadian citizens.

The Pro-Choice people justify this behaviour by stating that a woman has the right to have control over her own body. I agree wholeheartedly that she has the right to control **HER** own body. However, a woman's body has not, and never will include, the body of another individual which exists within her uterus. The fetus has never been considered to be an appendage of the woman. It is a separate organism altogether. The only connection it has with the mother is through the umbilical cord and the placenta through which it receives nourishment. If left unmolested, it will grow to be a normal, healthy, human baby.

The irony is that when abortion was removed from the Criminal Code, thereby permitting abortion on demand, the Prime Minister of Canada, Pierre Elliott Trudeau, and many of his senior cabinet ministers, were practising Catholics. Since abortion is forbidden by the Catholic Church, how did they reconcile their actions with the teachings of their Church?

For a number of years, the birth-rate in Canada has been declining steadily. At the present time, there are not enough babies being born annually to maintain our present population. This decline in the birth rate is most apparent in the province of Quebec. Over the past thirty years, the birth rate in Quebec has gone from the highest in the world to the lowest. Francophone couples average about one child per family.

Since the major fear of Francophones is the loss of their language and their culture (it used to be language, culture "and religion") this decreased birth rate does not make much sense. Our present Prime Minister is of the opinion that the only solution to the problem is to increase our population by increasing the number of immigrants. He does not believe that incentives which would encourage married couples to have more than one or two children would be of any benefit. He does not even mention the subject of abortion. That would be political suicide.

CHAPTER 10: YEAR TWO IN QUESNEL

Getting Some Experience Under My Belt

The physician can sometimes parry the scythe of death,
but has no power over the sand in the hour-glass.
Author Unknown

After spending a year in Quesnel, I was beginning to get the feel for it. The nurses at the hospital were very good. Half of them were young graduates, eager to learn and always trying to do their best. The more experienced ones were capable in all areas of nursing. They had the ability to handle anything calmly and with confidence. It was quite obvious that they loved the work they were doing. In spite of the relatively low wages, they were happy doing the work they loved.

By 1952, there were four doctors in town. Dr. Tompkins had decided that he preferred Quesnel to Vulcan and had returned to Quesnel. He was exceptionally good at looking after patients with emotional problems, besides being a very good surgeon. Dr. Appleby had joined us after doing a year's internship followed by a year of pathology at St. Paul's Hospital. He had done hundreds of autopsies during his year of pathology, but had decided that the specialty of pathology was not for him. Pathology's loss was our gain. He was invaluable in doing all of the autopsies that needed to be done. He was also a very careful and thorough individual when it came to the practice of medicine. I doubt if there was a more capable practitioner anywhere in Canada.

At that time, in spite of the fact that we had four doctors in Quesnel, we had designed a system of sharing emergency calls that was brutal. Each of us took turns being on call for emergencies. The doctor would go on call at 8 A.M. on Monday morning and be on call until 8 A.M. the following Monday.

Besides being on emergency call, he might have to be at the hospital before 8 A.M. in order to do elective surgery that had been scheduled, to assist someone else at surgery, or to give an anaesthetic for someone else. Then, after making rounds to see his patients in hospital, he would grab a quick lunch and rush to the office to begin seeing his patients in the office by 1 P.M. When he had finished seeing his patients at the office (usually around 6 P.M.) he would check with the receptionist to see if any patients had called requesting advice over the telephone or a house call.

If patients had phoned during the day, their names, phone numbers and messages would be put on a special spike at the receptionist's desk. The doctor on call would check for any messages and would usually make the calls before going home for dinner. At times, especially if there was an epidemic of influenza, it could be exhausting. Later on, we designed a system in which we were on call for shorter periods of time. Even then, we were usually kept very busy when we were on call.

I can recall one time when I was on call, I finished seeing patients in my office at 6:30 P.M. When I went to the front desk to pick up my messages and house calls, I had six house calls to make. That wasn't unusual because there happened to be an epidemic of influenza in town. However, before I could make those house calls, I was requested by the RCMP to do autopsies on three men who had been found dead in their car during a snow storm. Since the three corpses had the classical signs of carbon monoxide poisoning, those autopsies were probably the quickest ones ever performed in the Province of British Columbia.

On another occasion, I was asked by the corporal in charge of the RCMP office if I would meet him at the funeral parlor when I had finished seeing patients at the office. It was spring time and a man had just been found in the Fraser River. There was the possibility that he might be the same individual who had been reported missing the previous winter.

The corporal wanted my assistance in helping to identify this body. When I met the corporal outside of the funeral parlor, he had a small bottle of whisky in his hand. He said that I'd better have a good-sized drink before I entered the funeral home. I wasn't much of a drinker, but I didn't want to offend him so I took a swig. When we entered the funeral parlor, the odor that hit us was enough to make a person vomit. This fellow had been in the river all winter. His body was bloated and decomposed. My job was to amputate all of his fingers so they could be sent to the forensic lab of the RCMP in Regina in an endeavor to try to identify him. Why they needed all of his fingers I will never know. It didn't take me long to complete the job.

I got to know the RCMP officers in the town quite well. At times I would be called to court as an expert witness. The officers were cognizant of the fact that I was usually pressed for time and always took that into consideration. I would receive a telephone call at the office just before I was due to appear on the stand. I would drive immediately to the court house, give my testimony and be back in the office in a few minutes.

Another of the duties of the doctor on call was to examine prisoners in their cells prior to their being transferred to Vancouver by plane. The physician had to verify in writing that the prisoner did not have a communicable disease. It was against the law to transfer such a person on a public transit.

One Saturday evening I was phoned at home by the nurse who was working in the emergency room of the hospital. A workman had just been brought into the hospital from one of the small local sawmills. He was unconscious when he arrived at the hospital. Since I lived only a block from the hospital, I was able to get there in less than five minutes.

When I examined the patient, he was in a deep coma. Both pupils were dilated and fixed. He did not respond to any painful stimuli. There was a large hematoma (collection of blood) in the right temporal area. X-rays revealed that he had multiple fractures of the skull at the site of the hematoma. I phoned Dr. Peter Lehman, a young neurosurgeon at the Vancouver General Hospital. (It seems unbelievable when I think of it now, but there was not a single neurosurgeon on the staff of St. Paul's Hospital in the early 1950s.)

I explained the situation to Dr. Lehman and asked his permission to transfer the patient to Vancouver if arrangements could be made to have an emergency air force plane make the flight. Dr. Lehman advised me that he felt the patient was likely to die from the severe injury to the brain long before arrangements could be made to fly him to Vancouver.

He suggested that as a last resort we might attempt to relieve the intracranial pressure by making an opening into the skull. While the nurse shaved the hair at the operative site, Dr. Appleby and I scrubbed for what would be my first and only craniotomy. I made a large incision over the fracture site and freed the soft tissues from the underlying bone. Using a brace and a bit, I drilled a number of holes through the skull. These holes were joined using a Gigli saw so that we were able to remove a circular piece of the skull. The dura was then opened with scizzors. As soon as the dura was opened, brain tissue began to ooze through the opening. It reminded me of porridge boiling over.

It was obvious that the patient didn't have a hope. He expired within an hour of the surgery. I never was attracted to neurosurgery, but that episode convinced me that I was not designed for that particular specialty. At that time I remembered the words Dr. H.H. Hepburn, Professor of Neurosurgery at the University of Alberta, stated during the one and only lecture I can recall his giving us: *"The Creator causes general surgeons to experience the occasional failure in order to humble them. He allows the neurosurgeon to be successful only enough times to keep him from becoming discouraged"*.

One Sunday afternoon while I was enjoying a relaxing day at home with my family, the telephone rang. It was my next-door neighbour. She had just found her two-year old daughter with an open bottle half-full of aspirin tablets. The infant had obviously swallowed some of the tablets, but the mother had no idea how many tablets had been in the bottle.

I advised the mother to take the little girl to the emergency room of the hospital where I would meet her. Since there was no way of knowing how many tablets had been ingested, I had no choice but to wash out the stomach (gastric lavage). In order to do this, it was necessary to pass a large tube through the mouth and into the stomach.

In order to restrain the child, we had to "mummy" her (wrap her in a large sheet with only the head free). Swallowing a stomach tube is uncomfortable even for adults and causes them to gag considerably. For a young child it is quite a traumatic experience. In view of this, I advised the mother not to remain in the room during the procedure. We managed to complete the lavage without any difficulty and obtained several small pieces of the material that had been swallowed.

There are times, believe it or not, when the treatment is definitely harder on the doctor than it is on the patient. This was one of those times. However, my little patient did not show any signs of resentment towards me for the ordeal I had put her through. She continued to play with my young daughter, Brenda, as though nothing had happened.

A four-year old boy was brought in to see me because his parents noticed that he seemed to be having difficulty going up the stairs leading to the second floor of their home. Prior to this, he seemed all right to them except that perhaps he had been a little slower than his siblings in sitting up, standing and walking.

On examining him, there wasn't anything I could really put my finger on except that his calf muscles appeared to be unduly large and he had a certain waddling type of gait and tended to walk on his toes. I wondered if he might have some sort of condition affecting the skeletal muscles and suggested to the parents that it might be worthwhile to have him checked out in Vancouver.

I referred him to Dr. Peter Spohn, who arranged for tests such as electro-myography, measurement of serum enzymes and muscle biopsies. Investigation confirmed that he had a rare form of muscle condition called pseudohypertrophic muscular dystrophy. There was no known cause for this condition and no cure.

The family moved from Quesnel to Vancouver shortly after the diagnosis was made in the hope that some form of treatment might be available. He may have lived for a number of years, but eventually would have died from the disease, most likely due to failure of the muscles of respiration.

One of the problems I was faced with was both a medical one and an ethical one. I was called upon to attend a young man in his twenties who was bleeding quite profusely from the back of the nasal cavity. Although I had never had to treat a hemorrhage in this region, I knew what I had to do in order to get it under control.

The first procedure was to place a large, solid pack into the nasopharynx. The nasopharynx is the space at the back of the nasal cavity. After this pack was tightly in place, it was necessary to insert gauze packing from the front into both nasal cavities and to pack this tightly against the posterior pack. Theoretically, this blocked the whole nasal cavity and acted as a tamponade against the bleeding vessels. Most of the time this worked. Since the procedure was pretty uncomfortable to the patient, it was done under general anaesthesia.

The packing did slow the bleeding considerably but did not stop it completely. The patient continued to ooze through the packing so that eventually his blood loss became significant and alarming to me. The obvious solution to this, of course, was to replace the blood loss with transfusions of whole blood.

The only impediment to this was that the patient was a member of the Jehovah's Witness faith and thus refused to have any blood. As time went on, the situation became more and more desperate. Each day the patient became paler, his hemoglobin dropped further and he began to look like a ghost. After five days of slow but steady bleeding, the patient's wife persuaded him to allow me to transfuse him. I gave him four units of fresh blood, which not only improved his hemoglobin level and his color, but also had the effect of causing hemostasis.

After a couple of days of no further bleeding, I gently removed the anterior packs. When there was no recurrence of bleeding over a twenty-four hour period, I cut the posterior pack free and removed it. Again, there was no bleeding. It looked like whoever was watching over me had again come to my assistance.

This was my first experience in which there was an ethical conflict between the treatment I wished to carry out and the religious beliefs of the patient. Today, with the revolutionary advances in scientific medicine, doctors are being faced with ethical and moral decisions on a daily basis.

Should they keep the patient alive or allow him to die? Should they do everything they can to save the life of a tiny premature infant who has little hope of survival? Should they resuscitate a patient who has had a cardiac arrest, but is near death from cancer? Should they try to keep a newborn infant alive even though he has no brain or is so severely deformed that he will live for only a few hours or a few days? Should they transplant hearts into newborn infants or should they allow nature to take its course? Should they assist a patient to end his life if he has an incurable illness and wishes to die?

These questions, and similar ones, are being faced by doctors every day now. The decisions are not easy ones. Since the cost of medical care is also a factor, the solution is not only a medical one, but also an economic one.

One weekend, when I happened to be the only doctor in town, a rancher was brought to the hospital from the Nazko Valley. He had sustained severe lacerations of his left hand while he was cutting firewood with a chain saw. The lacerations extended across the palm of his hand, severing all of the tendons of the hand with the exception of his thumb.

Since there was no one available to give him an anaesthetic, I decided to repair the tendons using a form of local anaesthesia called a brachial plexus block. By inserting a long needle into the neck above the clavicle and directing it downward, the anaesthetic solution is injected in order to block the nerves which originate in the neck and extend downward into the arm. By means of this type of anaesthesia, it is possible to anaesthetize the whole arm.

A tourniquet can then be applied to the upper arm to allow the surgeon to work in a bloodless field.

I was able to locate the lacerated tendons and repair them in the usual fashion. The hand and arm were then put in a plaster cast for a sufficient length of time until healing had occurred. Fortunately, the wound did not become infected. Although the hand never returned to its normal condition prior to the injury, the patient did obtain a very functional hand considering the severity of the injuries.

I did a number of tendon repairs while I was in Quesnel, one of them on a two-year old boy who had cut the tendon of his thumb. I enjoyed this type of surgery very much. I can certainly appreciate why some orthopedic surgeons restrict their practices entirely to hand surgery. It is very enjoyable and rewarding work.

One afternoon I was called to the hospital to see a ten year-old boy who was a catcher on one of the little league ball teams. He had been accidentally hit on the head by one of the batters. He fell to the ground, but was unconscious for only a few seconds. I examined him carefully, but aside from a little swelling and tenderness of the left temporal area (the temple), there was nothing unusual. However, in view of the history, I admitted him to hospital for twenty-four hour observation. The nurses were instructed to check him every hour and to chart his pulse, blood pressure, breathing and the reaction of his pupils to light. They were advised to waken him every hour during the night.

About six hours after his admission to hospital, the nurse phoned me to say that the pupil of the left eye was slightly larger than that of the right eye and was not reacting to light as briskly as it had been. I went immediately to the hospital and confirmed the nurse's findings. This indicated to me that there was increasing intracranial pressure, probably due to bleeding from the middle meningeal artery. I phoned Dr. Peter Lehman in Vancouver, and described the situation to him. He arranged to have an air force plane flown to Quesnel in order to have the boy transferred to the Vancouver General Hospital. A few hours later, Dr. Lehman phoned to inform me that the boy had sustained an injury to the middle meningeal artery. He had done a craniotomy, removed the blood which had collected and clipped the bleeding artery. He would be sending the boy back to Quesnel in a few days.

I was called one day to one of the local sawmills. I had no idea when I started on the road what I was going to find when I arrived at the mill which was a few miles north of town. When I arrived at the mill, I was taken to the area where the pieces of rough lumber travelled along a conveyor belt after they had been cut by the saw.

Lying under the belt was a man who was in his middle thirties. He had apparently leaned over to move a piece of loose lumber from the belt and the bottom of his jacket had caught in the belt and drawn him into the flywheel. He was flung around so violently that he struck the ground, dislocating his neck. He had died instantly. This young man had a wife and four small children. This type of accident was not unusual among sawmill workers. Some people had labelled the sawmill industry "the maker of young widows".

On another occasion, I was called out to the Western Plywood Plant which was situated on the Fraser River just south of town. When I got there, I found a young man lying on the platform. He had been struck on the front of the right knee by a log. The blow caused the knee joint to bend severely backwards resulting in a compound fracture - dislocation of the joint. The popliteal artery could be seen pulsating in the wound. By some miracle, it had not been damaged.

We splinted the leg carefully and had him transported to the hospital. I phoned Dr. McConkey in Vancouver and arranged to have him transferred by air to St. Paul's Hospital. Dr. McConkey did an arthrodesis (fusion) of the knee joint. The workman ended up with a stiff right knee, but was very fortunate that he did not lose the leg. After he had completely recovered, he went to barber school and returned to Quesnel where he established a successful business. He also managed to play a pretty good game of golf.

One Sunday afternoon when I was on emergency call I was asked by patients of mine to see a friend who had been visiting from Prince George. He had stayed overnight with them and was now planning on driving back to Prince George. Shortly before he was preparing to leave, he began to develop slight chest pain. His guests were concerned about this pain and convinced him to see me before he left for Prince George.

He was a healthy-looking man in his mid-thirties. He had a history of having had a peptic ulcer, but otherwise had been very healthy and able to do hard physical work. The pain he described was mild, dull in nature and located behind the lower end of the sternum. It also extended into the area of the upper abdomen. Examination did not reveal anything unusual. In spite of his young age, I advised him that there was a possibility that the pain might be cardiac in origin. I advised him to defer his trip back to Prince George and instead to come with me to the hospital where we could keep an eye on him for a few hours and do a cardiogram. He insisted that he would be all right and that he wanted to head for home so that he could go to work the following morning.

His friends and I finally persuaded him to accompany me to the hospital. With that, I picked up my bag, started towards the door and asked him to follow me to the car. I hadn't quite reached the door when I heard a "thump" behind me. I turned around and saw that he had fallen to the floor. He didn't move. I ran over to him and saw that he was not breathing. I couldn't feel any pulse, there were no heart sounds, no blood pressure and his pupils were dilated and fixed. He had had a cardiac arrest.

Since this was in the days before external cardiac massage and cardio-pulmonary resuscitation had been described, there was nothing I could do for him (close-chest cardiac massage was developed in the early 60s). This young man had suddenly dropped dead and there was nothing that I could do. On that occasion, I experienced the most helpless feeling in my entire career. Subsequent autopsy revealed some atherosclerosis of the coronary arteries. He probably had had a sudden cardiac arrhythmia (irregular heartbeat) which caused instant death.

Of course today, CPR, carried out properly, could save the life of such a patient. Although there were times like this when very little could be done for the patient, there were other times when the life of the patient could be saved by proper treatment. This helped in a small way to compensate for our many inadequacies.

It's rather interesting how this husband and wife had become patients of mine. The husband had appeared one day in my office as an extra patient. He complained of a sore throat which he had had for a number of days. Since I had never seen him before, I did a complete history and physical examination which I was accustomed to doing. The only positive finding on physical examination was redness and swelling of his tonsils accompanied by swelling and tenderness of the cervical lymph nodes.

However, I was surprised when urinalysis revealed that he had sugar in the specimen of urine. Further investigation revealed that he was diabetic. His throat infection was treated with penicillin. His diabetes required insulin as well as a special diabetic diet.

I saw the wife for the first time in the emergency room of the hospital. She presented with sudden, severe, abdominal pain. Her history and physical examination indicated that she probably had an ectopic pregnancy. (An ectopic pregnancy is one in which the fertilized egg develops in one of the uterine tubes. As it develops, the tube ruptures causing severe bleeding into the abdominal cavity.) The diagnosis was confirmed by laparatomy (opening the abdomen) and the tube involved was removed.

One afternoon, the young minister of the United Church came to see me. He was a very dedicated, hard-working person who was devoted to the welfare of his parishioners. He explained to me that he had been having some peculiar symptoms periodically for about two weeks. He had noticed slight blurring of his vision, tingling of the face and numbness of his fingers. There had been the occasional headache. I examined him very carefully and thoroughly and could find nothing out of the ordinary.

I explained to him that I could find no evidence of any serious illness and that I suspected the symptoms might be due to the stress under which he had been working. I suggested that he take a couple of weeks off work and get away for a few days so that he could relax. He informed me that his parents lived in Ontario and that he would take my advice and visit them. Shortly after seeing him, I left town for a few days to visit my parents in Vancouver.

On returning to Quesnel, I learned that this patient of mine had taken a plane from Vancouver to

Toronto. On arriving in Toronto, he had suddenly lost consciousness. He was taken by ambulance to hospital where he had died in a matter of a few hours. An autopsy was carried out and revealed that he had died from a hemorrhage into a tumor of the brain.

Of course I was shocked to get this news. It drove home to me the fact that tumors of the brain can be present with very few symptoms and signs. Ruling out a brain tumor requires special tests. Today of course, the CAT scan and MRI are invaluable in detecting brain tumors. These were not available in the 1950s. The CAT scan was not generally available in B.C. until the 1980s and the MRI until the 1990s.

One morning, a patient of mine appeared in my office, quite upset. I had delivered her of a normal male infant one month previously. This was her fourth child so she was not the type to become alarmed for trivial things. She told me that the baby had been no problem until that morning when he began to have sudden crying spells. Nothing she had done could settle him down.

He was quiet when I began to examine him, but he soon began to cry quite loudly. While I was inspecting him in general, I noticed a small swelling in the right inguinal (groin) area. The swelling was soft and appeared to be a bit tender. It did not decrease in size nor disappear when I exerted gentle pressure on it. I felt that he had an incarcerated inguinal hernia and asked Dr. Avery if he would have a look at the baby.

Dr. Avery examined him and agreed with my diagnosis. We took him to the hospital and operated as quickly as possible. He did have an incarcerated hernia which was easily freed. Fortunately the circulation to the bowel had not been impaired so it was just a matter of freeing the bowel and closing off the hernial sac. If this diagnosis had been missed, the bowel would have become gangrenous, which very likely would have been fatal. This type of unexpected incident occurred quite frequently, making my practice a very exciting and rewarding one.

CHAPTER 11: AN UNUSUAL OBSTETRICAL COMPLICATION

And Other Surprises

*I used to wonder why people should be so fond of
the company of their physician, 'til I
recollected that he is the only person with whom
one dares to talk continually of oneself,
without interruption, contradiction, or censure.*
Mrs. Hannah Moore (1745 - 1833)

Connie and I were attending a dinner and dance at the local Legion one Saturday evening when I received a call from the hospital. While I was at the Legion, one of my maternity patients had been admitted to the hospital in labor. This was her fourth pregnancy. She was close to term and having regular contractions at the time of admission. A couple of hours after admission, the membranes ruptured and within a few minutes the nurse on duty was called to the labor room by the patient. The nurse was shocked at what she found and phoned me immediately.

I drove to the hospital as quickly as possible and went right to the labor room. I examined the patient and found that the umbilical cord had prolapsed and was protruding from the vagina. There was also one foot dangling from the vagina. There was no pulsation of the umbilical cord, which meant that the infant was dead. In view of this, there was no point in considering a cesarean section. Since the cervix was only partially dilated, it would have been dangerous to attempt vaginal delivery. I felt that I should wait until the cervix was fully dilated before attempting vaginal delivery.

To be on the safe side, I phoned Dr. Trowbridge, Chief of Obstetrics at St. Paul's in Vancouver, and explained the situation to him. He advised me to allow the patient to continue in labor and when the cervix was fully dilated, to deliver the infant by breech extraction. Fortunately, labor continued normally and when the cervix was fully dilated, I exerted traction on the foot which was lying outside of the vagina. I was then able to bring down the other foot and complete the delivery in the usual manner. There were no complications except that we had a dead baby. Although I had known how to handle the situation, until it was all over, it was a stressful event.

A woman in her early thirties appeared in my office one day for prenatal care. She had been married for a number of years and this was her first pregnancy. Examination revealed enlargement of the uterus consistent with about eight weeks of gestation. She was given the usual advice and advised to return in one month.

When she was seen one month later, she informed me that she had experienced no problems since the previous visit. Examination revealed the uterus to be the size consistent with about twelve weeks gestation. I saw her again in one month and, to my surprise, the uterus was now smaller than it had been during her previous visit. She had had no bleeding nor other problems since the last time that I had seen her. There had been no quickening (fetal movement) noticed at any time.

Since she was asymptomatic, I elected to observe her at weekly intervals. Over a period of about a month, the uterus gradually returned to its normal size and all symptoms and signs of pregnancy disappeared. I explained to her that I felt that she had experienced an uncommon condition known as missed abortion.

With this condition, a woman becomes pregnant, the pregnancy develops normally to a certain point, the fetus then dies for no apparent reason and over a period of time, the products of conception are absorbed. There is no bleeding, no pain, the signs of pregnancy disappear and the patient returns to her pre-pregnant state. The cause is unknown and there is no specific treatment required. Although this was quite a shock to the patient, she weathered the situation well and did not have any emotional problems as a result of it.

Although this case turned out all right, there were times when we were not so fortunate. One Saturday afternoon, I was called from the hospital by Dr. Avery to give an anesthetic for him. When I arrived at the hospital I found a young man lying on the operating table. He was unconscious. He had apparently been unloading a load of logs from his sideloader truck when the whole load of logs fell on him, crushing him.

He was brought to the hospital as quickly as possible, but was in severe shock when he arrived at the hospital. In spite of giving him whole blood transfusions, it was not possible to improve his condition to the point where it would be possible to carry out a laparotomy. Within a few hours of arriving at the hospital, he succumbed to the severe injuries. Subsequent autopsy revealed multiple intra-abdominal and intra-thoracic injuries.

During my time in Quesnel, there would be many young men in their prime who would be severely injured, sometimes fatally, while working in the small sawmills surrounding the village. There were a number of young married women, often with small children, who suddenly found themselves widowed.

Although we were often called upon to manage situations which belonged in the realm of the specialist, most of the time we managed to handle things ourselves. However, I recall one case in particular where the expertise of a trained surgeon was urgently needed.

Dr. Avery had been called to the emergency room to see a young boy who had fallen from his bicycle resulting in injury to the abdomen. Following his examination of the patient, Dr. Avery felt that the boy had probably sustained an injury to the spleen, a ruptured spleen. This results in considerable intra-abdominal hemorrhage. He knew, of course, that the treatment for this condition was splenectomy – surgical removal of the spleen. Although he had assisted at this surgical procedure during his surgical training, Dr. Avery felt that it would be too risky for him to do the surgery.

He therefore phoned Williams Lake and spoke to Dr. Ringwood, who was a certified surgeon practising in Williams Lake at that time. He explained the situation to Dr. Ringwood, who agreed to drive the seventy-five miles from Williams Lake to Quesnel in order to see the boy.

When Dr. Ringwood arrived at the hospital in Quesnel, he confirmed the diagnosis and agreed to do the surgery. With Drs. Avery and Tompkins assisting him, and with me giving the anesthetic, Dr. Ringwood carried out the splenectomy. The boy made an uneventful recovery. This boy's life had been saved by means of a careful history and physical examination by Dr. Avery. No exotic tests were needed to arrive at the cause of the problem.

The reader might be wondering how we managed to give blood transfusions to patients when there were no laboratory facilities at the hospital. Without a lab, it is not possible to determine the patient's blood type nor to cross-match it with stored blood. We solved this problem quite easily.

A couple of times a year members of the Red Cross would hold a blood-donor drive in the Village. Anyone who contributed blood during one of these clinics would have his name, phone number and blood type recorded. A copy of this list of donors was always kept at the hospital. If we needed blood for a patient, we would check this list and pick out one or more donors whose blood type was O, Rh negative.

This person was then phoned and informed that we had a patient who required a blood transfusion. He was asked if he would consider donating a pint of his blood. On no occasion do I ever recall a donor who was not very willing to donate his blood. This is the sort of response that is common in a small community. People are more than willing to help their neighbor.

When the donor arrived at the hospital, a pint of his blood was withdrawn in the usual manner. It was then given immediately to the patient. If more than one pint was required, we would contact two or more donors. Since the blood type was O, Rh Negative, the person was considered to be a universal donor and no cross-matching was required. So far as I am aware, there was never any reaction due to incompatibility of the blood. Perhaps we were lucky.

I was called to the hospital one evening to see a young married woman who had been admitted to the hospital a few minutes before the nurse phoned me. She was not a patient of mine, but was a patient of one of the other doctors who happened to be out of town at the time.

This young patient was in the third trimester (last three months) of her pregnancy. She was a primigravida (first pregnancy). The membranes had ruptured spontaneously prior to her admission to hospital and she was in active labor. The labor pains were strong and frequent at the time of my examination. It took her less than an hour from the time of admission to hospital until she delivered a live, premature, female infant. When we weighed the infant, we found that she was a mere two pounds, seven ounces.

Since we had no facilities for caring for such a tiny infant and no nurses with experience in caring for premature infants, it was apparent that she would have to be transferred to Vancouver if she was to survive. I phoned Dr. Peter Spohn and explained the situation to him. He advised me to look after the infant to the best of our abilities and that if she survived for twenty-four hours, he would arrange to have her transferred to Vancouver.

The nurses did a wonderful job in caring for the tiny infant. When I called Dr. Spohn the next day, he arranged to have an air force plane, equipped with an incubator and oxygen and accompanied by one of the nurses from the premature unit at St. Paul's, travel to Quesnel. The infant made the trip to Vancouver without incident, was cared for in the premature unit for a number of weeks and returned to Quesnel several weeks after her birth.

As a sequel to this story, in the summer of 1999, my wife and I were having lunch at the Mount Paul Golf Club in Kamloops one afternoon when a young man approached my wife and spoke to her. He had lived in Quesnel for a number of years before moving to Kamloops, and had recognized my wife as a former resident of Quesnel.

During the course of our conversation, I happened to mention that one of the many babies that I had delivered while I was doing general practice in Quesnel had weighed only two pounds, seven ounces. He informed us that he was related to this tiny patient, that she was now forty-three years old, was in excellent health and had three healthy children of her own.

In 1951, there were two pharmacists in Quesnel. Jim Kinley was located in the old Hudson Bay Building on the corner of Carson Avenue and Front Street. Len Barclay had a tiny store on Front Street near the old Rex Theatre. Len had just moved to Quesnel from Williams Lake where he had owned a drugstore for a number of years.

It wasn't long before both of them built new stores on Reid Street. In a matter of months, Jim acquired an assistant, Alf Spencer, who took over the store when Jim became ill. Jim began to have trouble with his memory which deteriorated over a short period of time.

I can recall many times phoning a prescription to him and having to repeat it several times before he would get it straight. He went to see the experts in Vancouver and they came up with the diagnosis of "atrophy of the brain".

Today, we know the condition as Alzheimer's Disease. When Jim's condition became severe enough that he was unable to work, Alf took over the job on his own. In time, he brought in a classmate of his to share the work load. The store was subsequently renamed Spencer-Dickie Drugs.

CHAPTER 12:
ANESTHETIC COMPLICATIONS

And Other Problems

Any fool can take off a leg. It takes a surgeon to save one.
George Ross – Montreal Surgeon

During my ten years of practice in the Cariboo, I gave hundreds of anesthetics. I began by using open-drop ether using an ether mask for general anesthesia requiring relaxation of the abdominal muscles. I progressed from this to the use of a modern anesthetic machine allowing me to use nitrous oxide, cycloproprane, oxygen and muscle relaxants. Intravenous pentothal was used for short, general anesthesia requiring no relaxation. Local anesthesia, nerve blocks and spinal anesthesia were used whenever possible.

During those ten years, I can recall three anesthetic complications. The first one involved a patient who was having a hydrocele repair. (A hydrocele is a cyst located in the scrotal sac.) As soon as the local anesthetic had been injected, the patient had a grand-mal seizure which lasted for only a few seconds. He recovered from this completely with no apparent ill-effects.

The second patient was being given a brachial-plexus block for surgery on his hand. Again, as soon as the anesthetic had been injected, the patient had a convulsion which lasted for only a few seconds. He also recovered completely from the seizure. In both of these cases, the anesthetic solution had probably been injected accidentally into a vein.

The third patient was a one-year old infant who was having a general anesthetic for the surgical treatment of an incarcerated hernia. Near the completion of the surgical procedure, the patient suddenly stopped breathing. I immediately checked his pulse and found none. There were no heart sounds audible and no carotid pulse. His pupils were dilated and fixed. All of these signs were indicative of cardiac arrest.

Artificial ventilation was carried out but was not successful in restoring the action of the heart. Since closed-chest cardiac massage had not been described at that time, (cardiac massage was first described in the literature in the late 60s and early 70s) there was nothing further that could be done.

The loss of a young patient is always a terrible tragedy, especially when it occurs during a surgical procedure. I fretted about this for quite some time, but finally came to realize that this was not benefiting either me or my patients. It had always been a worry for me to give an anesthetic to an infant, but after that episode, it was more stressful than ever.

Prior to the time of obtaining an anaesthetic machine, there were two surgical procedures for which I did not enjoy giving the anaesthetic. One was the removal of tonsils and adenoids and the other was total dental extraction. In both of these conditions, there could be considerable bleeding, which was always a worry due to the possibility of obstruction of the airway.

When I was using open-drop ether for these procedures, there could be a fair amount of stress involved. For tonsil and adenoid surgery, I started the anesthetic using vinethene (vinyl ether), which put the patient to sleep in a few seconds. I then switched to ether and continued with this for several minutes in order to get the patient into a deeper plane of anesthesia.

After one tonsil had been removed and the bleeding had been controlled, it was not unusual for the patient to start to wake up. It was then necessary to renew administration of the ether until the patient was deep enough for the surgeon to remove the other tonsil. If there was active bleeding at this time, it presented a real problem to the anesthetist because of the possibility of blood obstructing the airway. He had to alternate between suctioning the blood from the throat and pouring the ether.

One of the local dentists preferred to do his total extractions under general anesthesia when he was going to fit the patient with dentures. Instead of removing three or four teeth, allowing the wound to heal, then repeating this a number of times, he preferred to admit the patient to hospital and remove all of the teeth at one time.

After I got the patient deep enough with ether, he would extract the teeth as quickly as he could, trying to complete the job before the patient started to awaken. He didn't bother to use any sutures in order to control the bleeding and hasten healing, so there was usually considerable active bleeding. If a tooth happened to get broken off at the gum margin during the procedure, thereby requiring more time to extract the root of the tooth, the patient would start to awaken. With considerable bleeding going on, this could create some tense moments.

When we started to use the gas machine, and to intubate patients, we had much better control of the airway. This allowed the surgeon to take his time in getting the bleeding under control without having to worry about the patient waking up.

In 1952, Dr. Appleby had left St. Paul's Hospital in Vancouver to come to Quesnel. Instead of having a morgue with all of the modern conveniences in which to carry out autopsies, he now had a morgue which was located in a small wooden shack behind the hospital.

One winter day, I was waiting to help him with an autopsy. It was so cold that we decided to warm up the building by lighting a fire in the small pot-bellied stove. While we were waiting in the hospital for the morgue to warm up, the stove got so hot that it started a fire in the building. We managed to extinguish the fire quickly, but not before the corpse had sustained some superficial burns.

However, we completed the autopsy without further interruptions.

Years later, when we moved into the new hospital, Dr. Appleby had all of the equipment and conditions he had become accustomed to while doing autopsies at St. Paul's.

Although I was busy enough as it was in my practice looking after Homo sapiens, it was not unusual for me to be asked to see a sick or injured animal. Since there was no trained veterinarian in town, I could hardly refuse such a request.

On one occasion, I was asked by a woman if I would make a house call to see her dog. The dog had developed a severe rash.

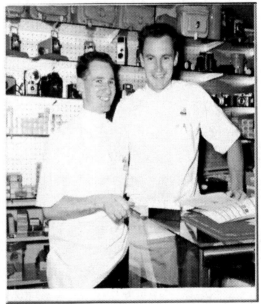

PHOTO 42 [Alf Spencer and Don Dickie -two of the local pharmacists]

She not only asked me if I would make a house call to see the dog, but if I would send the bill for my services to her health-insurance company. She had

M.S.A. insurance. When I informed her that I thought it would be stretching things to consider her dog as a member of the family, she was a bit upset.

Today, the way many people treat their pets, I sometimes have the feeling that the pets are not only considered to be members of the family, but are given more attention and care than the children.

I recall another case in my veterinarian practice when a gentleman appeared at the front door of my home. Although he had had no formal training, he considered himself to be the local veterinarian. He asked me if I would look at a dog that he had in his car. He thought that the dog might have cancer of the rectum.

When I examined the dog, I found a large, fungating tumor protruding from the anus. Although I had never seen a tumor of the rectum in a dog, I felt quite confident in advising him that he was correct in the diagnosis and that there was not much that could be done in the way of treatment.

It wasn't long before Alf Spencer and Don Dickie were being asked for their opinions concerning treatment of various illnesses and injuries in animals. Within a period of a short time, they became quite knowledgeable in veterinarian medicine and surgery. For many years they supplied a real service to the local ranchers, not only with regard to the medical treatment of various conditions but also in the surgical management of many injuries.

CHAPTER 13: THE ROYAL ALEXANDRA HOSPITAL

A Wonderful Place to Learn Obstetrics

The rapid increase of knowledge has made concentration in work a necessity.
Specialism is here and here to stay. The desire for expert knowledge is now so great that there is a grave danger lest the family doctor should become a relic of the past.

Sir William Osler – 1892

After being in Quesnel for a number of months, I made the decision that general practice in a small town was the type of work I enjoyed. The work was interesting, challenging and rewarding – not financially, but spiritually. Most of the people were young. All of the people were friendly. Of course there were periods of disappointment, sorrow, feelings of inadequacy and frustration, but these were compensated for by the successes and the feeling of being needed and appreciated. Most of the people were satisfied with the quality of medical care they were receiving. They appeared to appreciate that we were trying to do our best.

We had four full-time doctors in Quesnel, all of them good practitioners and compatible with one another. Each one had his area of expertise. We formed a partnership and made plans for the construction of a new office building. We shared emergency calls and assisted each other in surgery. Everyone shared the work load equally. Whenever we were in town, we did our own obstetrics.

We were all young, full of energy and enthusiasm for our work. Dr. Avery was an excellent surgeon, showed good judgment and could be depended upon when we had difficult or unusual surgical problems. We would not have been able to do many of the surgical procedures we did, had it not been for his expertise.

I had not been in Quesnel for very many weeks when I realized that there was one area of deficiency in my training for this type of country practice. I had not had enough training in obstetrics so that I could feel comfortable and competent.

Obstetrics is an area in which things can go bad very quickly and unexpectedly. Although it may be true that having a baby is a normal physiological process most of the time, there is always the possibility of a sudden, unexpected and unforeseen complication. This can turn a happy, quiet, memorable event into a nightmare. Since the nearest obstetricians were in Kamloops, we were required to look after any and all obstetrical complications without the help of a specialist. This was a heavy burden and created a great deal of stress at times.

Fortunately for me, in 1953 the Royal Alexandra Hospital in Edmonton, most often referred to as the "Alex", was in the process of building a new maternity hospital. I applied for a one-year residency position in obstetrics and was very fortunate to be chosen from several applicants.

When I informed Dr. Baker that I had done this, he was happy to hear of my decision. He gave me a letter of recommendation to present to the head of the department of Obstetrics. I still have this letter. A copy is reproduced at the end of this chapter. I felt very honoured to have received this letter from Dr. Baker and have kept it as one of my treasured possessions.

When I started at the Alex, I was the assistant resident in obstetrics and gynecology. The resident, Percy Glady, had just completed a year of obstetrics at St. Louis, Missouri and was now in his second year. As a point of interest, Percy had been a classmate of Lyon Appleby's at Queen's University. Half way through the year, Percy became ill, an event which required him to drop out of the program at Christmas.

In one way, this was a benefit to me. In another way, it was not so good. I was now the only resident in obstetrics and the only one on the obstetrical service, with the exception of the interns, who spent one month each on the service as part of their rotation. Since I was the only resident, I had the choice of surgeries I wished to assist at and the deliveries I wished to attend.

However, it also meant I would be very busy and have more responsibilities. I was on call at the hospital every second night for the remainder of the year. This was very rewarding educationally, but extremely fatiguing. It also meant that I had very little free time to spend with my wife and young son.

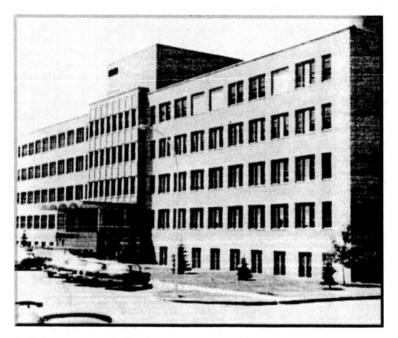

PHOTO 43 [Photo of Royal Alexandra Maternity Hospital in Edmonton, Alberta]

The new hospital was beautiful. There were one hundred beds, four labor rooms, two delivery rooms and a large operating theatre, which was used only for caesarean sections. Our section rate for the year was two percent. The acceptable caesarean section rate at that time was two to four percent. Anything over four percent was considered to be bad obstetrics. We practised very conservative obstetrics.

At the present time, in some hospitals, it is not unusual to have a section rate of twenty-five percent.

There are many reasons for this; the expectation and demand by the mother of getting a healthy baby, careful fetal monitoring, repeat caesareans, the fear by an obstetrician that he might be sued if he delivers a damaged infant, and more aggressive treatment of complications of labor. At times, the attitude appears to be "if in doubt, operate".

During the twelve-month period that I spent at the new obstetrical hospital, we delivered over five thousand babies, more than any other hospital in Canada. Since I was anxious to get as much experience as possible, I personally delivered several hundred babies. With this volume of obstetrics, I was able to see a large number of abnormal obstetrical patients who were bleeding before, during and after delivery, patients with toxemia of pregnancy (pre-eclampsia and eclampsia), many requiring forceps assistance, many with difficult and prolonged labors and many other unusual conditions. I was able to use the different types of forceps which had been designed for specific purposes.

Bleeding which occurs during a pregnancy is designated by different terms depending on the period of the pregnancy and the cause of the bleeding. Threatened abortion refers to vaginal bleeding which occurs during the early months of pregnancy. For no apparent reason, the patient begins to bleed. The bleeding may range from slight, intermittent spotting, to severe hemorrhage. Sometimes this bleeding stops spontaneously and the pregnancy continues on to term without any further problems. At other times, the bleeding continues until the fetus and placenta are expelled from the uterus. When this occurs, bleeding usually ceases over a few days. At times, when the bleeding is severe enough, the patient is advised to stay in bed until the bleeding ceases or the fetus and placenta are expelled. Spontaneous abortions are usually considered to be nature's way of getting rid of an abnormal fetus – the so-called blighted ovum.

Abruption of the placenta refers to premature detachment of a normally-implanted placenta. For some unknown reason, the placenta suddenly separates from the wall of the uterus at a specific site with bleeding occurring between the wall of the uterus and the placenta. Sometimes there is bleeding into the muscular wall of the uterus. There is usually severe pain, vaginal bleeding and tenderness at the site of detachment of the placenta. If the detachment involves a large segment of the uterus, there can be severe bleeding into the uterine wall, external hemorrhage, death of the fetus due to loss of blood supply, and even death of the mother from shock. Abruption of the placenta is frequently associated with severe toxemia. Abruption of the placenta is always to be considered an obstetrical emergency.

Placenta praevia refers to the situation in which the placenta is located in the lower region of the uterus, at or near the cervix. As the cervix progressively dilates during labor, the placenta begins to separate from the wall of the uterus at the region of dilatation. This is a very serious complication of pregnancy and is accompanied by bleeding which can be horrendous. Any bleeding which occurs during a pregnancy can be serious and is always a worry, especially if it occurs during the last three months of pregnancy.

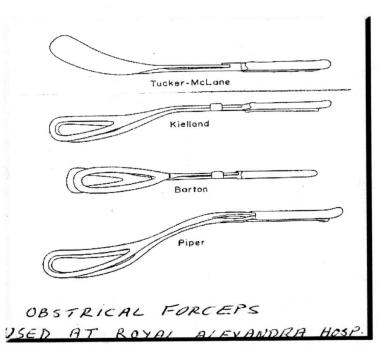

PHOTO 44 [Drawing of various forceps]

The most common forceps used were the Maclean forceps and the Tucker-Maclean. These were used when the patient required a little assistance with the delivery of the head of the infant. The Tucker-Maclean was also used by some obstetricians to rotate the head of the infant from the posterior or transverse position to the anterior position. The

Kielland forceps was a specially designed forceps which was used only to rotate the head from the transverse to the anterior position. The Barton forceps was also specially designed to rotate the head from the transverse to the anterior position. It had an anterior blade which was hinged in order to make it easier to apply to the head. The Piper forceps was designed specifically for the delivery of the after-coming head in a breech delivery. I had the opportunity of using all of these forceps and in becoming proficient in their use. I was able to utilize this knowledge many times after I returned to Quesnel.

Pre-eclampsia (also known as toxemia of pregnancy) was, and still is, one of the dreaded complications of pregnancy. It occurs during the last three months of a pregnancy and is commonly associated with the first pregnancy. With this condition, the patient's blood pressure becomes elevated, there may be edema (swelling) of the face, hands and feet, there may be headache and disturbance of the vision. The cause of this condition remains a mystery. The most effective treatment is delivery of the fetus.

However, this can create problems if the infant is not mature enough to survive. If the patient is near term, induction of labor is the treatment of choice. If the condition progresses, the patient may have convulsions (eclampsia) and other more serious complications such as hemorrhage into the retina, cerebral hemorrhage, or even death. I saw a number of pre-eclamptic patients and learned how to manage this condition properly. However, the outcome is never assured to be favorable and it always remained a worry.

I learned that there are different ways of dealing with various problems in obstetrics and that no one way is the only or correct way. For example, when I was on the obstetrical service at St. Paul's Hospital during my year of internship, I had been taught that when a patient starts to bleed in the first few weeks of a pregnancy (threatened abortion) that it was better not to do a pelvic examination for fear of causing more bleeding and for fear of increasing the risk of abortion. We were taught to put the patient in bed, elevate the foot of the bed and hope that the bleeding would stop. However, at the Alex, the teaching was to insert a speculum into the vagina and examine the cervix carefully. Often we would find a piece of placenta stuck in the cervix. When this was removed with a forceps, the bleeding would stop.

Sometimes, prior to the delivery of the head of the infant, it is necessary to enlarge the opening of the vagina by doing an episiotomy (making an incision with scissors). At St. Paul's we were taught to do a medio-lateral episiotomy (make the cut from the midline outwards). The reason for this was to prevent the episiotomy from extending into the rectum. At the Alex, we were taught to make a median episiotomy (down the centre). If the episiotomy happened to extend into the rectum during the delivery of the head of the infant, it was a matter of recognizing this and repairing it properly. The advantage of the midline episiotomy was that it was less painful to the patient during the healing period and it also healed more quickly. I preferred to use the median episiotomy for the rest of my career in obstetrics.

As I mentioned previously, I saw many unusual and interesting patients during the year that I spent at the Royal Alexandra Hospital in Edmonton. I would like to mention a few of these patients.

As a rule, after the delivery of an infant, it is only a matter of a few minutes before the placenta separates spontaneously from the wall of the uterus and is expelled. On rare occasions, the placenta fails to separate from the uterus spontaneously. This is referred to as a placenta accreta. When this occurs, it is necessary for the obstetrician to insert a hand into the uterus, very carefully free the placenta from the wall of the uterus with the side of the hand with a cutting motion, and remove the placenta with his hand. I had the opportunity of doing this on two occasions. It was a useful maneuver to be familiar with.

On another occasion, an obstetrician who had been trained at the Cleveland Clinic was faced with the situation where the infant's head was in the transverse position. This was not unusual and I'm sure he had dealt with it before dozens of times. Doctors who were trained at the Cleveland Clinic were taught to use nothing but Tucker-Maclean forceps. The teaching was that if you couldn't rotate the head of the infant with Tucker-Maclean forceps, you couldn't do it with any other forceps. After attempting to apply the forceps to the head of the infant, he found that he was unable to get the anterior blade into position properly. After several attempts, he declared that we would have to take the patient to surgery to do a caesarean section.

I asked him if he would let me try to use the Kielland forceps, and to my surprise, he said "*go ahead*". He didn't think I'd be able to do it. I had no difficulty in applying the Kielland forceps because it had been designed specifically for this situation. I applied the forceps and rotated the head to the anterior position without any difficulty. I then removed the forceps and completed the delivery using the Tucker-Maclean forceps. Both of us had learned something from this. He learned that the Tucker-Maclean forceps could not always be relied upon for this situation. I learned that the Kielland forceps was a very useful forceps for this particular problem.

Another time, I was in the case room to assist with the delivery of a woman who was having her ninth baby. Ordinarily, you would expect that this would be a simple, straight-forward procedure. However, the obstetrician found that the baby was lying sideways in the uterus (transverse lie). He was a very experienced practitioner. He decided he was going to deliver the baby by what is known as a version and extraction. He inserted his hand inside the uterus, grasped one foot of the infant, pulled it down, and delivered the infant as a breech. The maneuver looked very easy and slick.

However, within a few seconds of delivery, the mother's blood pressure dropped, her pulse became rapid and thready, and she stopped breathing. Attempts by the anaesthetist to revive her were unsuccessful. In less than a minute, she was dead. Autopsy revealed a tear right across the lower end of the uterus which included both uterine arteries. She had died from massive hemorrhage.

A twenty-two year old woman was admitted to hospital at thirty-six weeks gestation. Her blood pressure was very high, she had edema of both feet and there was protein in her urine. She was treated conservatively in the usual manner with strict bed rest, sedation and magnesium sulfate. She was considered to be a severe pre-eclamptic. Before we were able to reduce her blood pressure to a reasonable level, she began convulsing (eclampsia), lost consciousness and died. Autopsy revealed that death was due to a massive cerebral hemorrhage.

Another young woman was admitted to hospital with pre-eclampsia. Her blood pressure was very high and she had moderate edema of her feet and hands along with proteinuria. Following bed rest and sedation, her blood pressure dropped considerably. After several hours, we started induction of labor using a pitocin drip intravenously. I sat with her with my hand on the abdomen in order to feel the uterine contractions.

I regulated the rate of the pitocin drip in order to bring on regular uterine contractions. When the cervix had dilated sufficiently, the membranes were stripped and ruptured. The pitocin drip was continued until the cervix was fully dilated. The patient was then delivered with the assistance of forceps. However, during the labor, she had sustained several small hemorrhages into the retinae of both eyes resulting in considerable loss of vision in both eyes.

One evening I was called to the case room by the nurse to assist in the delivery of a patient of Dr. Stephen Parlee. I had considered him to be the most competent obstetrician in Edmonton. I was waiting in the delivery room while Dr. Parlee was scrubbing in the other room.

Suddenly, the patient began to hemorrhage. The blood ran out of the vagina as if someone had suddenly turned on a tap. I called Dr. Parlee to come into the delivery room right away. He came in immediately, did not bother to put on a gown nor gloves, reached into the vagina with his hand, grasped the foot of the baby and delivered it as a breech. The patient was given intravenous pitocin to cause the uterus to contract and the placenta to separate and be expelled. This patient had a marginal placenta praevia. When the cervix became fully dilated, part of the placenta separated, causing massive bleeding.

If Dr. Parlee had not been there and attended to the problem immediately, the patient would have bled to death in a very short time. This was the most frightening thing I ever experienced in all the years associated with obstetrics. This served to reinforce my belief that serious problems can develop very quickly in obstetrics. If these cannot be dealt with properly and quickly, the patient could be lost. In view of this, in my opinion, there is no place for home delivery in this day and age, in this country. The risk might be minimal, but is it worth taking if you don't have to do so?

After I decided that Dr. Parlee was the best obstetrician in Edmonton, I asked the nurse to call me whenever he had a delivery. In time, he allowed me to do many of his deliveries while he stood by.

On one occasion, I was waiting for him in the case room when he poked his head through the door and asked me what was the position of the baby. I replied that the head was in the posterior position. To my surprise, he told me to go ahead and rotate the head and deliver the baby.

I applied the Tucker-Maclean forceps, rotated the head, removed the blades, reapplied them and delivered the head. To my surprise and embarrassment, the head came out "face to pubis". I had rotated the head from the "anterior" to the "posterior" and delivered it in that position. I expected Dr. Parlee to be pretty upset with my mistake, but to my relief and surprise, he merely laughed and said "*Now you can call yourself an obstetrician*".

There were a few obstetricians in Edmonton who did most of their work at other hospitals, but would come over to the Alex for the occasional delivery.

One of these doctors, who was an excellent obstetrician, was quite a showman. At times, when there was a student nurse or a medical student in the delivery room, he would put on a show just for their benefit. When the patient was just about ready to deliver spontaneously, he would shout to the head nurse "bring the tongs quickly". The nurse would go out of the room and return in a few seconds with a tiny pair of wooden forceps. These were replicas of the first type of forceps designed a couple of hundred years ago. They resembled a pair of wooden spoons and were about ten inches in length. He would apply these "tongs" to the infant's head, brace his left foot against the delivery table and pretend to pull for all he was worth. Of course, the infant's head would appear spontaneously with the next contraction of the uterus assisted by the push of the mother. It was quite a show. No matter how many times I saw this performance, I couldn't help bursting out in laughter every time I witnessed the exhibition.

On one occasion when I was assisting this same obstetrician with a caesarean section, he decided to see how fast he could deliver the infant. He asked the nurse to time him from the time he made the incision in the skin until the baby was delivered. At the word "go", he made a deep incision which went through the skin, underlying muscle and the uterus. He quickly enlarged the incision in the uterus with his index fingers and delivered the infant. The whole procedure took a matter of a few seconds. It was quite a display of showmanship.

There was one thing, however, which detracted from the performance. When we looked at the infant, he had a small superficial incision on his scalp! Fortunately, it wasn't deep enough to require sutures. I wasn't with him when he explained the wound to the mother.

While we were in Edmonton, Connie, my wife, began to have moderately severe, intermittent pelvic pain. She was seen by Dr. Parlee, who found that she had an ovarian cyst the size of an orange. He scheduled her for surgery in order to remove the cyst. She was admitted to the hospital the afternoon before the day of surgery.

On the evening before surgery, Dr. Parlee visited her and did a pelvic examination in order to determine whether there had been any change in the size of the cyst since his last examination. To his surprise, the cyst was no longer present. Apparently, it had been a follicular cyst which had ruptured spontaneously since his first examination. Surgery was then cancelled.

On June 4th, 1954 our son Phil turned three. Since Connie was anxious to have more children, she began to worry that something might be wrong as we had used no contraception. Dr. Parlee examined her, found no abnormalities and arranged to do a hysterosalpingogram. This procedure consists of injecting lipiodal, a contrast medium into the uterus and uterine tubes and checking by means of the fluoroscope and x-rays to see if the dye passed through the uterus, through the uterine tubes and spilled into the pelvic cavity. This enables the gynaecologist to determine whether there is any obstruction of the passages. As it turned out, everything was clear.

It wasn't long after having the salpingogram that Connie became pregnant. There probably had been a slight obstruction of the uterine tubes due to a previous mild inflammation following a miscarriage she had had in 1952. The dye flowing through the uterine cavity and uterine tubes under slight pressure, had probably broken down the adhesions.

After my year of obstetrics, Dr. Allen Day, head of the department of obstetrics, tried to encourage me to continue on in the program in order to become an obstetrician. This would have meant two more years of training. However, I still felt that I wanted to return to general practice in Quesnel. I came close to going to Trail instead of back to Quesnel, because I had received an offer to go to the C.S. Williams Clinic to do obstetrics there. I had a great year at the Royal Alex, one I shall always remember. The training I received there would be invaluable to me when I returned to the Cariboo.

Copy of letter of recommendation written for me by Dr. Baker in 1953 prior to my going to the Royal Alexandra Hospital in Edmonton for a one-year residency in obstetrics:

To Whom It May Concern:
I hereby certify that Dr. Leonard Maher has been an associate of mine in the Quesnel Clinic. I consider him a man of outstanding ability, very conscientious,

kind to his patients and a most pleasant personality
to work with.
Gerald R. Baker, FRCS
Quesnel, B.C.
20th March, 1953

CHAPTER 14: RETURN TO THE CARIBOO

A brand-new Clinic and Hospital

Equanimitas is the ability to stay calm in the face of disaster.

Sir William Osler

While we were in Edmonton, Dr. Baker had died. Since his health had been failing at the time I left Quesnel, it was no great surprise when I learned he had passed away. That was the end of a wonderful man, a friend and a legendary pioneer of the medical profession in British Columbia. The world would be much better with more men like him. He was an ardent fisherman and hunter, but above all he was a caring and competent doctor.

When I returned to Quesnel in 1954, the Quesnel Clinic building was being rebuilt by Eric Sargent. Most of the original bungalow was retained, but a considerable addition was under construction. We obtained permission from the hospital board to relocate our offices temporarily into the old nurses' residence located just south of the old hospital. This was an old building where single nurses had their living quarters. My temporary office was a tiny room just large enough to accommodate an examination table and a couple of chairs. We were like sardines in a can. We remained in these quarters for several weeks until our new office building was completed.

We renamed the building The Avery Clinic in honour of Dr. Frank Avery.

In the new building, we had an abundance of space. The ground floor consisted of a large waiting room, an area for the receptionist and the filing cabinets where the records of the patients were stored, a small room for the office manager, Warren Woodhurst, and a small emergency room which was used for suturing wounds, changing dressings, applying plaster casts and other minor procedures. We also had a small lab where we could check the urine of patients and examine specimens with a microscope. Each of the four doctors had an office and an examining room. We also had hot running water with which to wash our hands! There was a full basement with a gas furnace and a large room which we used as a lunch room and library. This was a tremendous improvement over our previous quarters.

Construction of a new hospital was begun in 1954 and completed in 1955. The hospital was located on Front Street just south of the old nurses' residence. It was a two-storey building with all of the modern facilities for a hospital of its size. On the first floor was the main entrance, the walls of which were covered by murals depicting some of the events in the life of Dr. Baker. The main office, x-ray department, laboratory, emergency room and surgical suite were also on this floor. There were several rooms for patients, a nursing station where the records of the patients were located along with their medication and a small room in which the doctors dictated the histories of their patients and their operative reports. The second floor contained two labor rooms, a delivery room, a nursery for the newborn infants, a nursing station and several rooms for patients.

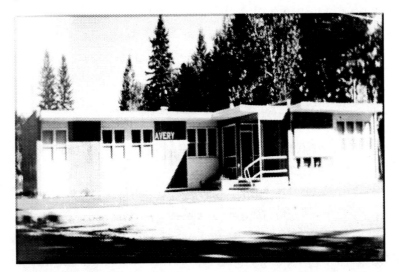

PHOTO 45 [Photo of the Avery Clinic on Front Street]

With the completion of the new office building and hospital, along with a certified x-ray technician, Bob Bushnell, as well as a laboratory technician, we had definitely gone from rags to riches.

In order to utilize our x-ray facilities to the maximum, Dr. Appleby arranged to spend a couple of weeks in the x-ray department at St. Paul's Hospital where he learned to carry out barium studies of the esophagus, stomach, small and large intestines. This allowed for considerable improvement in the investigation of patients with gastro-intestinal problems.

Along with the large operating room, we had a modern up-to-date anaesthetic machine which would enable us to give safer anaesthetics. However, since none of us had any real training in the use of one of these gas machines, the question arose as to who would be the first to get this training. Since no one showed any real enthusiasm for anaesthesia, I volunteered to go down to St. Paul's Hospital to get the training.

I arranged to spend one month on the anaesthesia service at St. Paul's. Most of this time was spent with Dr. Mary Mate, a certified anaesthetist and a classmate of Dr. Appleby's. Dr. Mate was an excellent teacher. She was organized, methodical and strict. She showed me enough in one month to enable me to give satisfactory, safe anaesthetics using the new machine. I learned how to intubate patients, how to use nitrous oxide and cyclopropane, and how to use muscle relaxants.

On my return to Quesnel, I had no problem in using the new gas machine and in teaching the other doctors what I had learned. Dr. Appleby showed particular interest in anaesthesia and became very competent in this area. Before long, he and I were giving almost all of the anaesthetics.

It wasn't long after my return to Quesnel before my obstetrical training in Edmonton was put to the test. One Saturday afternoon, when I was on call, Ann Gagnon phoned me from the hospital.

There was a patient of Dr. Appleby's who had been in labor for a number of hours and was now thought to be ready for delivery. The nurses were unable to contact Dr. Appleby because he was out of town at the time.

From my home I ran down the back road to the hospital and hurried to the delivery room. After scrubbing and gowning, I examined the patient, who was a primigravida (first pregnancy). Examination revealed that the infant was in the breech position. As the contractions continued, one foot appeared at the opening of the vagina.

I grasped the foot and pulled it down. With continued contractions, I delivered the rest of the infant, except for the head. I lifted the feet and arms of the infant, and asked the nurse to hold them up for me so that I could apply Piper's forceps to the head. I got the first blade on without difficulty, but when I attempted to apply the second blade, the infant's head turned sideways, thus making it impossible to apply the second blade. I had to take the feet from the nurse and allow the baby to drop downward in order to permit the head to rotate back into proper position.

Repeating the maneuver a second time, I was able to apply the forceps and deliver the head without difficulty. All of this probably took less than two minutes. However, at the time, it seemed like an eternity. When the baby was weighed later, she weighed more than nine pounds.

During a breech delivery, it is wise not to rush things, but it is important to complete the delivery as quickly as possible once it is started. If the infant starts to breathe before the head has been delivered completely, he might become anoxic, thereby causing damage to the brain.

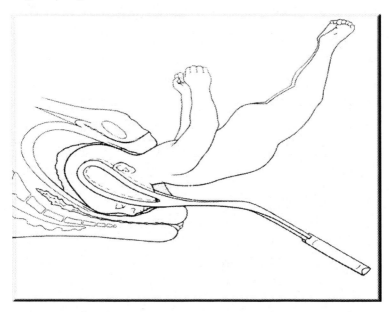

PHOTO 46 [Diagram showing delivery of after – coming head of breech with Piper forceps]

The delivery of a breech during a first pregnancy can be hazardous because the mother does not have what is referred to as "a proven pelvis". There is no way of knowing with certainty whether the baby's head will be small enough to pass through the birth canal.

Today, if an infant is found to be in the breech position at the time that a primigravida is expected to go into labor, the delivery is usually carried out by caesarean section. The obstetrician is unwilling to risk the possibility of damage to the infant. I can't say that I blame him for adopting this attitude. The delivery of a primip.breech can be a very stressful event. As you can imagine, I was very thankful for having learned how to use Piper's forceps, otherwise, this large infant may have been damaged or lost.

Not long after returning to Quesnel, we moved from the little house we had been renting on Front Street into a larger home which we had purchased on Walkem Street. We were still located one block from the office and one block from the hospital. I was spoiled by being so close to my work. The house was less than one thousand square feet in area.

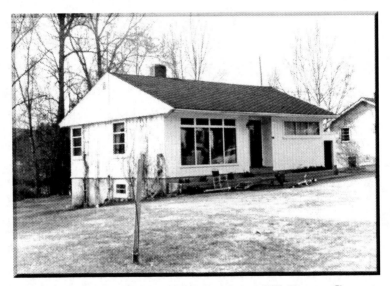

PHOTO 47 [Photo of home on Walkem Street, Quesnel]

The purchase also included a 60 – foot lot beside the house. The total cost was $12,000. Interest rates were about 4%. The location of the house was ideal for me. The hospital and the Clinic were less than a block from the house. The house had a kitchen, a small dining room off the kitchen, a living room with a fireplace, a bathroom and two bedrooms. There was a full basement with a furnace that burned sawdust. There was a separate area in the basement which was used to store sawdust and a small bedroom. There was also a tiny garage attached to the house. What made the location of the house even more pleasant was that it was situated on the east bank of the Fraser River. When we moved into our new home, we thought that we were in heaven.

Our next – door neighbours were Alex and Gertrude Fraser. Alex was the mayor of Quesnel for about twenty years. After retiring as mayor, he became the M.L.A. for the Cariboo, a position he held for many years until his death. He was Minister of Highways for about ten years. During his tenure as Minister of Highways, the Coquihalla Highway was built.

My wife Connie and I developed a close relationship with Alex and Gertrude. Our son Phil, who was three years old at the time, became very fond of Alex. He used to help Alex mow the lawn with his toy lawn mower.

Alex was brave enough to invite me to play lead for his curling rink in spite of the fact that I had never curled and knew nothing of the game. When I was young, we considered curling and golf to be games played by older people. We preferred games with plenty of action. When I was young, and until I completed university, the sports I participated in were softball, baseball, football, hockey and boxing. Alex's rink consisted of me as lead, John Diakiw (one of the local plumbers) as second, Jack Allison (the postmaster) as third and Alex as Skip. I never did improve my game for two reasons; I was often called to the hospital for an emergency or delivery just before starting a game, or part – way through a game. I also did not have any time to practise which is important if one is to improve in any sport. In spite of that, Alex and the other members of the rink never complained about how poorly I played.

It was a very sad day for us when we received word that Alex had developed cancer of the larynx (vocal cords). Alex was advised that the only treatment for his condition was a total laryngectomy (removal of the voice box) plus removal of all of the lymph nodes of the neck (known as a radical neck dissection). Since this would mean the loss of his voice, he was very reluctant to have the surgery. After speaking to the Otolaryngologist who was caring for Alex, I phoned Alex to advise him that the surgery was his only hope for a cure. He decided to go ahead with the surgery and asked me if I would be present in the operating room during the procedure. I was invited to assist with the surgery but decided only to observe it. Unfortunately, the operation prolonged Alex's life for only a few short months.

Subsequent to his death, the Alex Fraser Memorial Bridge in Vancouver was named in his memory. This bridge crosses the Fraser River from Delta to Annacis Island.

It wasn't long before I had a very busy obstetrical practice. I was soon delivering dozens of babies a year. This is a large volume for a general practitioner. I tried to live by the motto of the specialty of obstetrics - *Primum non nocere*, or, first do no harm. I practised very conservative obstetrics, which included forceps and caesarean sections when they were needed.

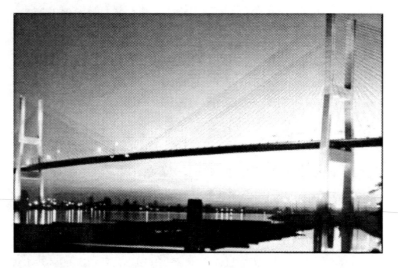

PHOTO 48 [Photo of Alex Fraser Memorial Bridge, Vancouver]

For most deliveries, I used no anaesthetics. If I thought I was going to need an episiotomy, I used a form of local anaesthesia called pudendal block. If I needed to do a forceps rotation and delivery, I used a form of spinal anaesthesia known as a saddle block. With the patient sitting up, a small amount of anaesthetic solution was put into the spinal canal. This anaesthetized the outlet of the vagina, the rectum and the area between them, known as the perineum. In this way, I could deliver the patient without causing any pain. An episiotomy could be done, if necessary, and sutured later without any discomfort to the patient. For breech deliveries (rear-end first), I preferred to have the patient fully co-operative and so avoided any type of anaesthesia. I did not use general anaesthesia for any of my deliveries. I used spinal anaesthesia whenever a caesarean section was required.

It has been said that a good obstetrician needs to practise masterful inactivity and watchful expectancy. Knowing when to let nature take its course and when to assist the patient requires good judgment. This comes from not only having adequate training but a lot of experience. It is probably the most important attribute of a good obstetrician.

Soon after returning to Quesnel, Connie got pregnant for the third time (she had lost one pregnancy at about six weeks gestation in 1952) and we had a second son, Dan. This was followed by two more pregnancies so that we were soon to have four children: Phil, Dan, Brenda and Paul.

Besides being very busy with my medical practice, I participated in a number of community activities which cut into the time I had to spend with my family. During the winter, I helped to coach one

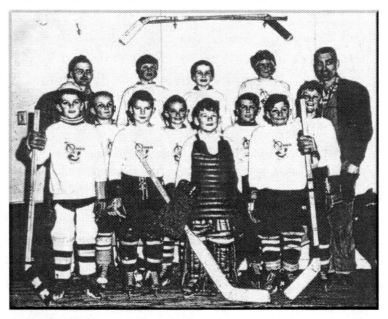

PHOTO 49 [Photo of the hockey team which I helped to coach. Author is in the back row next to son, Phil]

of the minor hockey teams. The boys were aged six to ten. Since my son Phil was starting to play hockey, I felt that I should help in some way. We had a lot of fun and stressed learning and enjoying the game rather than winning at all costs.

In the winter time, I had a small skating rink on the lot beside our house. Our children and the other children in the neighbourhood had a lot of good times on this small rink. Phil, Dan and Brenda, along with some of their friends, learned to skate on this rink. Once a year we had a hockey game between the boys and their fathers, which was always an exciting time.

I believe that today a lot of the enjoyment of hockey (and other sports) has been taken out of the game. Many of the coaches and parents, especially the parents, think that winning is the most important thing. They seem to have forgotten that the primary purpose of any game is to have fun. I think it would be much better for the boys and girls if things were not so organized and tournaments were kept to a minimum. There should be more fun and less stress when it comes to children's sports and other activities.

I also looked after a group of about a dozen boys, ages six to ten, as the "Akela" of a cub scout pack. We met every Friday evening from 6 – 9 p.m. in a small log cabin just north of the telephone building. With the help of Bert Gagnon, a planer-mill foreman, we had installed a new floor in the old cabin. All of the lumber was donated by Art Stack, the owner of the mill which was located at Kersley.

We spent most of the evenings playing games and instructing them in what it meant to be a good cub. Fortunately, I was assisted by a young fellow named Steve Piskorak, who was a great help to me. I looked forward to spending Friday evenings with these boys because they were so happy and full of enthusiasm. It really doesn't take a lot of expensive equipment to keep a group of young boys happy. I was also a member of the Lion's Club, although I missed more meetings than I attended. John Harvey, the president, did not consider me to be one of the outstanding members of the club, I am sure.

I was also one of the few male members of the St. Ann's Church choir. We used to hold our practices at Loretta Avery's home. However, I missed a lot of these practices also. Loretta was an excellent pianist.

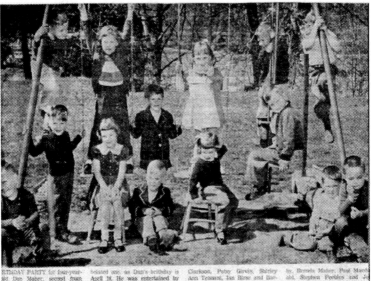

PHOTO 50 [Newspaper clipping from the local newspaper, the *Cariboo Observer*, relating to a birthday party we had for our son Dan. Two of my other children, Brenda and Paul, are also in the picture, as are Leslie and Len Appleby, two children of Dr. Appleby]

My burgeoning practice also had repercussions for my family. The wife of a country doctor does not have an enviable life. When the phone rings at two in the morning, it does not awaken only the doctor. Sometimes it also wakens the children. There were many times when plans were made to attend a picnic, go to a movie or a dance only to have to cancel things at the last minute because of an emergency. Many times, just when the family was ready to sit down to Christmas or Thanksgiving dinner, there was a call to the case room.

Because I was so busy with my practice, I have to give full credit to Connie for raising the children. Although I spent as much of my spare time with the family as was possible, most of the family matters became the responsibility of my wife. When we were in medical school, we were taught that the patient must always come first. Today's students and young doctors are not as strict about the call of duty. They spend more time with their families and allow more time for recreation and relaxation. This certainly helps to improve the family situation for the doctor and his family.

While my obstetrical practice was busy, I also attended upon other medical matters. In the autumn, it was not unusual to see patients with poliomyelitis. On some occasions, there would be epidemics in which several patients would contract the disease. Most of these patients had non-paralytic polio and would merely have symptoms which were similar to those of influenza. The occasional one would

215

develop weakness of various muscle groups, usually arms and legs. On rare occasions, patients might have involvement of the muscles of respiration or the cranial nuclei. When this happened, we referred these patients immediately to the department of communicable diseases of the Vancouver General Hospital. The reason for this was that if respiration became quite difficult, or impossible, the patient would have to be put on a respirator. Prior to these patients leaving the hospital we did a tracheotomy to ensure there would be no problem with obstruction of the airway during flight.

One evening while we were having dinner, the telephone rang. Connie answered it and informed me that it was Harold Johnson, our local chiropractor. He wanted to ask me about a patient of his, a young boy whom he had been treating for pain and stiffness of the muscles of the neck. He had just seen the boy, who told him that whenever he drank liquid the fluid would come back up through his nose. This new symptom had Harold baffled, but I knew immediately what the problem was without even seeing the boy. He had bulbar polio with paralysis of the muscles of the soft palate. I advised Harold of this and told him to have the boy taken to the hospital immediately and that arrangements would have to be made to refer him to Vancouver. This was definitely one condition that chiropractic manipulation would not cure.

The year that I had spent in Edmonton there was the worst epidemic of polio on record. When patients developed difficulty with their breathing, they were taken to a special unit at the Royal Alexandra Hospital, where they were put on respirators. They were called "Iron Lungs" in those days. There were twenty-two iron lungs in all at the hospital. These respirators were large boxes which enclosed the whole patient, except for his head. They always reminded me of coffins. When all of the respirators were in use, if a new patient was admitted with respiratory distress, the disease would have to be allowed to take its course. Often the patient died.

During this epidemic, our son Phil, who was two years old at the time, developed fever, vomiting and diarrhea. We were concerned enough at the time that Connie arranged to have him seen at the emergency department of the General Hospital by Dr. Porier, a paediatriciain. Dr. Porier examined him carefully, but could find no evidence of involvement of the nervous system. In retrospect I felt that he probably had non-paralytic polio. It caused considerable anxiety for us at the time, but fortunately he recovered from the illness in three or four days.

Every intern and resident had to spend a month in this unit helping to care for these patients. It was very depressing. I was the only doctor in training who did not have to spend time in the unit. Since I was on obstetrics, there was a fear that I might carry the disease to the mothers or the infants. I was therefore exempted, for which I was grateful. Since the development of the Salk Vaccine, followed by the Sabin Vaccine in the early 1960s, resulting in almost universal immunization, poliomyelitis is a rare event in Canada. There are not many medical students in Canada today who have ever seen or will likely ever see a patient with acute poliomyelitis. However, within the past few months a recently recognized complication of polio has appeared. It is called post-polio syndrome. Anyone who has had polio in the past is at risk for developing this condition. Post-polio syndrome is a slowly progressive, degenerative disorder that can appear years after the initial infection. The patients may experience fatigue, muscle and joint pain, muscle weakness, breathing difficulties, problems with swallowing and depression. So far, there is no specific treatment for the syndrome.

One afternoon I had a married man in his mid-thirties come in to see me because he and his wife had decided that they didn't want any more children. He asked me if I would do a vasectomy for him. I had to advise him that sterilization was illegal in Canada. About two weeks later, he returned to me and told me that he had had a vasectomy performed in Bellingham. He gave me a condom which contained some of his semen and asked me if I would check it for him. After checking the specimen under the microscope, and observing no sperm to be present, I informed him that the surgery appeared to have been successful. This was the one and only time that a patient had requested a vasectomy. I did not have any female patients request tubal ligations.

Today, in Canada, many women are having difficulty getting pregnant. In the 1950s in Quesnel, infertility was not a great problem. It appeared that all a man had to do was to hang his trousers over the railing at the foot of the bed and his wife became pregnant. Since the "pill" had not yet been discovered, there were some pretty large families.

I recall one married couple who were in their late thirties and were anxious to have a child. In view of their age, they were not eligible to apply for the adoption of a baby through the regular channels. They asked me if there was any possibility that I might be able to help them. I told them that I would do what I could. At the time, I had a classmate who was practising obstetrics in Rossland. I phoned him to inquire whether there was any possibility that he might be able to find a newborn infant for this couple. He said that he might be able to help.

A few days before Christmas, my classmate phoned the couple in Quesnel. He advised them that he had just delivered a young girl, that she was not married, and wished to put the baby up for adoption. The couple drove immediately to Rossland to pick up the baby. What a Christmas present that turned out to be!

However, I did have the occasional woman come in to see me because she had been married two or three years, had been anxious to start a family and had been unable to conceive. These women were usually in their mid or late twenties and in good general health. Besides doing a complete history and physical examination, I went through a fairly simple routine in my investigation of infertility.

One of the first things to determine was whether or not her husband was producing normal sperm. In order to do this, I had the woman do one of two things. I made another appointment for her to come into the office and requested that she and her husband have intercourse as close to the time of the appointment as possible. When she came into the office, I had her remove her underclothes and lie on the examination table. I then inserted a vaginal speculum and removed a small quantity of the fresh semen. This was examined immediately under the microscope to determine whether or not there were motile sperm present. If there were active sperm, I assumed that the husband was probably all right. If there were no sperm present, it would indicate that this was likely the problem.

If this type of arrangement was not possible, I requested that the couple have intercourse as close to the time of the appointment of the wife as possible. The husband was advised to use a condom so that a specimen of semen could be obtained for examination. If the specimen of semen was normal, I instructed the wife to check her temperature at the same time each morning and to plot the results on graph paper. This was done in order to determine whether or not she was ovulating (producing an ovum) each month. If it was determined that normal ovulation was occurring, then it was necessary to find out whether or not the uterine canal and uterine tubes were open or blocked. This was determined by doing a hysterosalpingogram. A solution of lipiodol was injected into the cervical canal of the uterus while the patient was examined in the x-ray department with the fluoroscope. If the passages were patent, the dye would flow freely through the uterine canal and uterine tubes and spill into the pelvic cavity. If there was an obstruction, the dye would reveal the site of obstruction. The advice to the patient would depend upon the results of the investigation. Of course, this is an oversimplification of the subject of conception and infertility.

Many of the medical matters that came to my attention took on personal significance given that I was a doctor in a small community. In cities, people tend to associate mainly with those who belong to the same socio-economic group, and therefore, have a very narrow range of friends. When viewed from this perspective, life can be much more interesting and rewarding in a small town than it is in a city where everyone appears to be in a hurry, is not particularly interested in his next-door neighbour, but tends to confine himself to his own little group of friends. I always had the feeling that my patients appreciated what I was doing for them and were thankful to have me as a personal friend. My maternity patients in particular seemed satisfied that I was doing my best to look after their needs and that of their children.

One of the more intimate relationships that my family and I developed began early one Sunday morning in July, 1958. I was called to the emergency room to see a patient who had just driven from Barkerville with his two sons. He was a forty-five year old ophthalmologist who lived and practised in Oregon City. He and his two sons were on their way home from a camping trip. When they were within a few miles of Quesnel, the father, Dr. Henry Schlegel, began to have chest pain. He managed to keep driving until he reached the hospital. When I saw him, he was having a moderate amount of pain, slight shortness of breath, nausea and weakness. His blood pressure was normal, but his pulse was rapid and weak.

I felt that his pain was cardiac in origin so I started him on oxygen and gave him small doses of morphine intravenously until he was free of pain. An electrocardiogram revealed changes which were in keeping with myocardial ischemia (insufficient blood supply to the heart muscle). Subsequent testing confirmed that he had indeed suffered a myocardial infarct. I placed him on the acceptable treatment at that time, which consisted of absolute bed rest, heparin for a few hours intravenously and dicumarol. He responded well to this regimen.

My wife had his trailer and car moved to the vacant lot beside our home so that the boys could be close to their father. Henry Schlegel remained in hospital under my care for a month. During that time the boys ate with our family, were free to come and go as they pleased, and slept in their trailer. They were able to visit their father at the hospital whenever they pleased. Henry was very pleased with the care he received, and in particular, the quality of the nursing care. He developed a friendly relationship with one of the nurses in particular, Ann McKenzie, who had lost her husband a few years previously from leukemia.

When the time arrived that I felt it was safe for him to leave hospital and return to Oregon, Connie drove him and the two boys to the airport. Ann had made arrangements to take off a few days from work the following week and was planning on visiting them. We received a phone call from Henry the following day advising us that they had arrived home safely, and thanking us profusely for our kindness to him and the boys.

Two days later, I received a phone call from one of Henry's partners advising me that Henry had died suddenly from a massive cerebral hemorrhage. It was a terrible shock to all of us, especially to Ann. A few days later, I received a parcel in the mail from Oregon City. It contained a Burberry raincoat and a letter. The coat was a new one that I had recently purchased. When Henry had admired this coat and asked where he might purchase one, I gave it to him as a going-away present the day he had left Quesnel. The letter was from Rick, his older son. In it, he expressed his gratitude for all that we had done for his father, himself and his younger brother. He also stated that he believed the cerebral hemorrhage sustained by his father might have been due to an overdosage of the anticoagulant being used by the attending doctor. And so, in a matter of a few days, a relationship which would have lasted for a number of years I am sure, was brought to a sudden end.

However, life goes on and I continued to get busier and busier with each passing day. My family was growing and I was spending less and less time with them due to a prodigious caseload.

One day a young lady in her mid-twenties phoned me at the office to inform me that she had begun to have brisk vaginal bleeding. She was around the sixteenth week of her first pregnancy. I had seen her previously at about the eighth and twelfth weeks of her pregnancy and things seemed to be quite normal at those visits, except that during the latter visit, the uterus appeared to be larger than usual for that period of gestation. I noted that there was a possibility of a twin pregnancy (ultrasound was not being used at this time during pregnancy). I advised the patient to have her husband take her to the hospital immediately and that I would be there when she arrived.

When I examined her abdomen, I was surprised to find that the uterus was considerably larger than I would have expected for this stage of her pregnancy. She had felt no movement of the infant, and there were no heart sounds audible. Vaginal examination revealed fresh blood in the vagina. The cervix was closed. I treated her in the usual manner with bed rest and mild sedation. The following day, the woman began to have strong uterine contractions with considerable pain. Within a short time she passed a large mass which resembled a bunch of grapes. I had never seen such a thing before, but I knew that this mass was a hydatid mole, a tumor which arises from the placenta.

Hydatid moles are tumors which develop from the placental tissue to form large masses as vesicles resembling grapes. They are usually benign, but can undergo malignant change. Most doctors will never see one of these during a practice extending over thirty to forty years.

I phoned Dr. Trowbridge, head of the department of obstetrics at St. Paul's Hospital in order to get his advice on the management of this problem. He advised me to do nothing in the way of surgical intervention so long as the patient did not develop alarming bleeding. I was fortunate in that she had expelled the mole completely and did not bleed much more than any person who had had a spontaneous abortion. She remained in hospital for a few days until the bleeding had ceased altogether. I then arranged for her to be seen by Dr. Trowbridge for investigation and any further treatment which might be needed. Fortunately, no further treatment was needed.

However, at another time one evening I was called to the emergency room to see a woman who had come in because of heavy vaginal bleeding. This patient was forty-two years of age, separated from her husband and living with a boyfriend. She thought that she was about three months' pregnant. Within a few hours, she passed what was quite obviously a hydatid mole. The bleeding gradually subsided and ceased entirely over a period of a few days. I advised her that she should be seen by a specialist, and that she should allow me to make arrangements for her to go to Vancouver in order to see a specialist. I felt that a hysterectomy should be seriously considered. After talking this over with her boyfriend, she was adamant that she did not want to have a hysterectomy. Her boyfriend was anxious to have a family. She remained in hospital until the bleeding had stopped, after which she was discharged. I arranged an appointment for her to be seen in the office for follow-up in two weeks. She did not keep her appointment.

Several months were to pass when I was called to the hospital to see a patient who had been brought in semi-comatose. I recognized her as my previous patient. Within a few short hours, she expired. Autopsy revealed that she had developed a choriocarcinoma of the uterus and that the tumor had metastasized (spread) via the blood stream to the brain. This was a malignant tumor which had probably developed from the mole she had expelled a few months previously.

Often less than common matters were to arise during my career. I had delivered a young lady of her first infant, a boy, following a normal pregnancy. The day she was discharged from hospital, I had circumcised the infant at the mother's request. The following day, the mother phoned to advise me that there had been continual oozing of blood at the site of the circumcision. I advised her to bring the baby to the office as soon as possible so that I could see him. When I saw him at the office there was slight bleeding from the wound. The bleeding would stop for a short time after pressure had been applied, but would resume within a few minutes. In view of this, I suspected that he might have a disorder affecting the coagulation of his blood. I asked the mother if she had any relatives who had bleeding problems. She informed me that she had a younger brother who had suffered from episodes of bruising and bleeding all of his life. In view of this, I suspected the infant might have hemophilia and arranged to have him seen by Dr. Peter Spohn.

Investigation revealed that the infant had a deficiency of factor VIII in his blood resulting in Classic Hemophilia. I was to see this boy periodically during the remaining years of my stay in Quesnel. He was seen for bleeding episodes due to slight trauma to various areas; the lip, palate, various joints and the kidney. He was seen when he needed to have a dental extraction. During each episode of bleeding, he was given fresh frozen plasma, which always brought the bleeding under control because it supplied him with the necessary factor VIII.

To add insult to injury, I looked after this boy's mother during her second pregnancy resulting in another son. As luck would have it, this boy also had a deficiency of factor VIII. In spite of the enormity of the problem, this mother coped exceedingly well whenever she was faced with a bleeding episode of one of her sons. I will always admire her ability to remain calm and to deal with the situation.

As an epilogue to this tale, I was stunned one evening, around the year 1997. I was watching the CBC News when a young man in his thirties appeared on the screen. He was making his way to Ottawa to plead the case for hemophiliacs who had contracted AIDS as a result of receiving blood contaminated with the HIV virus. This young man was in the final stages of AIDS. He was the same individual I had delivered years ago.

One morning when I was on emergency call, a woman phoned to ask if I would make a house call to see her baby who had a bad cold. Whenever I was asked to make a house call to see a sick infant or child, I tried to make the call as quickly as possible because I could never be sure of how sick the child might be. Some mothers were inclined to panic at the least little thing, while others did not call the doctor unless the child was seriously ill.

When I arrived at the house, I was astounded to find such a sick infant. The mother had not appeared to be particularly worried when I spoke to her on the phone. The infant's color was not very good. She had suprasternal and subcostal indrawing, characteristic of upper airway obstruction. Her temperature was 103 degrees F. I advised the mother that this baby was seriously ill and required an immediate tracheotomy. I had her get into my car with her baby and drove to the hospital immediately.

While Dr. Appleby administered the anaesthetic, Dr. Avery and I did an immediate tracheotomy. The baby's breathing improved dramatically following surgery. We placed her in a croupette (oxygen tent) with a high humidity and started her on antibiotics. She recovered completely in a few days and then we were faced with the task of removing the tracheotomy tube. I tried on three occasions to remove the tracheotomy tube, but each time, the infant went into immediate respiratory distress, forcing me to re-insert the tube. After the third failure, I phoned Dr. Peter Spohn and explained the situation to him. He advised me to send the patient to Vancouver where they would extubate her fairly quickly (so he thought).

It took them a whole month to wean the infant from the tracheotomy tube. I didn't feel like such a failure after receiving that news. Although this story had a happy ending, the same cannot be said for the following patient with a similar problem.

I was asked by Dr. Avery to see a two-year old infant that he had admitted to hospital. When I examined him, he was having considerable difficulty with his breathing and his color was poor. His lungs were clear. I felt that he had acute laryngo tracheobronchitis and that he should have a tracheotomy. I gave the anaesthetic while Drs. Avery and Tompkins did the tracheotomy. We placed the baby in a croupette with a high humidity, and started him on intravenous antibiotics. Although he seemed to improve initially, his condition worsened and he died a few hours after the tracheotomy had been done. The following day, I assisted Dr. Appleby with the autopsy. The trachea and the right and left main bronchi were completely obstructed with thick mucus. The patient had died from asphyxia.

After we had been in the new hospital for a couple of years, we applied to have the hospital evaluated for accreditation. A committee of experts came to Quesnel and went over the hospital from top to bottom. The records of the patients, operative reports, laboratory procedures, anaesthetic techniques, X-ray examinations, autopsies, surgical procedures, maternity care, and everything pertaining to the operation of the hospital were evaluated and found to be in order. This meant that we were doing things to their standards. We were all very proud. The G.R. Baker Memorial Hospital was the first hospital in British Columbia north of Kamloops to be granted full accreditation. This was considered to be a real honor to the medical, nursing, laboratory, X-ray, and administrative departments.

Chapter 15: GENERAL PRACTICE IN THE 1950s COMPARED TO TODAY

More Art, Less Science

The heroic adventures of today are part of tomorrow's ordinary medical care.

Author Unknown

General practice (now referred to as *FAMILY PRACTICE*) is that branch of medicine which provides primary and continuing care to patients irrespective of their age, sex or type of problem. Family doctors enter into a long-term relationship with their patients. They have full knowledge of the patient's family history, past medical history, present illness, medications being taken, allergies and other factors which are important in managing the health of the patient. The office visits of their patients provide an excellent opportunity for health education as well as the early detection of disease.

A high percentage of illnesses can be managed by the family doctor. Since he lives in the same community in which he practices, he is able to gain valuable knowledge of the working and living environment of his patients. Pre-natal, post-natal and well-baby care are important parts of his practice. A large percentage of babies born in Canada are delivered by the family doctor. Obstetrics remains an important part of family practice and should not be relegated to midwives. The family doctor is better qualified than anyone to provide comprehensive care to the patient.

I was disappointed when I learned recently that only twenty-four percent of family doctors in British Columbia are practising obstetrics. I assumed that the reasons for this were the increased rate of malpractice insurance charged to doctors doing obstetrics, the fear of being sued by the patient if there were any complications during or after the delivery, the failure to get a "perfect" baby, or the relatively poor remuneration for the care.

I was surprised to learn that the major reason for family doctors not wanting to do obstetrics was that it interfered with their "lifestyle". They did not want to be called out of the office, get up at night, nor have to be available on weekends or holidays in order to deliver babies. The family doctor who is unwilling to do obstetrics is missing out on one of the most enjoyable and rewarding parts of family practice. He is also losing a golden opportunity to establish a wonderful rapport with the patient and her family.

There have been innumerable changes in the practice of medicine over the past half century. To mention all of these would require a book in itself. One of the changes which I recall vividly occurred in the early sixties. It involved the manner in which doctors wrote their **PRESCRIPTIONS**. For centuries, the Apothecaries System of Measurements had been used. In this system, liquid medications were measured in minims, drams, and ounces. One minim was equivalent to one drop, one dram was equal to one tablespoonsful, and one ounce was about two tablespoonsfuls. Solid medications or those in powder form were prescribed in grains or parts of a grain. Peculiar abbreviations were used when writing these prescriptions.

In the early sixties, there was a sudden change to the Metric System. This change occurred while I was doing post-graduate work at the Medical College of Virginia in Richmond, Virginia. The first prescription I wrote for a hospital patient was returned to the nursing station by the pharmacist along with a note which said "If you want this prescription filled, write it in the Metric System." Needless to say, I felt stupid and embarrassed. It didn't take me long to "think Metric". The Metric System is easier and simpler. The mistake many people make is converting from one system to the other.

Many **TREATMENTS** are available today which were not in the 1950s. In 1953, I delivered an Italian immigrant of a male infant after a normal pregnancy and labor. The infant was perfectly healthy at the time of birth and also when I examined him at six weeks of age. Fours months after delivery, the mother returned to see me because the baby had become irritable and was not feeding well. It was readily apparent that he was severely jaundiced. His urine was dark in color and his stools were clay-colored. His liver was enlarged.

These findings were suggestive of some form of biliary obstruction. I referred him to Dr. Peter Spohn in Vancouver for investigation. He was found to have congenital atresia of the bile ducts (the bile ducts were obstructed). At that time, there was no treatment for this condition. The infant lived until he was two years old. He became more and more jaundiced, emaciated and finally died. It was difficult to watch the slow death of this couple's first-born infant. Today, surgical treatment is available for conditions such as this.

An eight-year old boy was brought in to see me because his mother had noticed that he had a slight limp at times. The limp would occur for no apparent reason. There was no history of any injury. He did not complain of any pain unless he had been unusually active, but even then, if he lay down for an hour or two, the pain would disappear. Examination revealed some limitation of the movement of the right hip joint. There was slight atrophy (wasting) of the muscles of the thigh, buttocks and calf. X-rays of the hip joint showed changes of the head of the femur which were suggestive of a condition known as Legge-Perthe's Disease.

I referred the patient to Dr. McConkey, orthopedic surgeon, who confirmed the diagnosis. The cause of this condition is unknown, although many theories have been put forth. Various forms of treatment have been tried, but there is still controversy as to what is the best. Dr. McConkey elected to treat him conservatively with bed rest, non-weight bearing exercises and ambulation. The outcome of treatment can never be anticipated with certainty. Some patients heal with no residual effects, while others sustain severe and permanent damage to the joint. At that time, nothing could be done if the patient sustained total destruction of the joint. Today, total hip replacement can be carried out resulting in a well-functioning joint with complete freedom from pain. Many other joints are also now being successfully replaced.

A remarkable change which has occurred over the years involves **IMMUNIZATION** against infectious diseases. When my children were infants, they were inoculated by the public health nurse in order to protect them from contracting diphtheria, typhoid fever, pertussis (whooping cough) and tetanus. At one year of age, they were vaccinated for small pox. In the early 1960s, they were given Salk Vaccine when it became available. This was to protect them against poliomyelitis (polio), also known as infantile paralysis.

Today, infants and children are immunized against diphtheria, pertussis, tetanus, polio, Rubeola (measles), Rubella, mumps, hepatitis B and Haemophilus influenzae. Meningococcal Vaccine is also available for protection against meningococcal meningitis, but is not supplied free of charge by the Public Health Department. Since 1975, vaccination against smallpox has no longer been carried out, as this disease has been eradicated.

As I mentioned earlier, the doctors in the Avery Clinic used to take turns being on call for emergencies. In the smaller towns and villages of British Columbia, some sort of arrangement similar to this probably still takes place, otherwise a family doctor would have no free time. However, even when I was not on call for emergencies, whenever Connie and I went to a movie, hockey game, baseball game, dance, or any other public event, it was not unusual for someone to buttonhole me in order to discuss some problem he, his wife, or one of his children might be having.

For a number of years, in the larger cities, the hospitals have had *EMERGENCY-ROOM PHYSICIANS.* These are medical doctors who after graduating from medical school have taken two or more years of special training to prepare them to treat emergencies. They are experts in dealing with all types of emergencies, medical and surgical. They may see the patient, prescribe the appropriate treatment and allow the patient to go home, advising him to see his family doctor at a later date for follow-up.

If necessary, the emergency-room physician may have another specialist see the patient while he is at the hospital. The specialist may arrange emergency surgery or admit the patient to hospital for treatment. As you can appreciate, the emergency room physician has the effect of decreasing the volume of work required to be done by the family doctor after regular office hours, weekends and holidays.

A major change which has occurred in recent years is the increasing use of so-called *DAY SURGERY*. Prior to this, patients who were to have surgery were almost invariably admitted to hospital the afternoon before the day of surgery. Any necessary investigative work would be ordered and both the surgeon and anaesthetist would examine the patient that afternoon or evening to ensure the patient was in good enough condition for the surgery. Surgery would be carried out the following day. The patient would be discharged from hospital in one or more days, depending upon the surgical procedure which had been carried out and his postoperative condition.

For a number of years now, however, when the surgeon books the patient for surgery, he indicates that the procedure is to be done in Day Surgery. Any investigative laboratory work would already have been carried out between the time the patient was seen by the surgeon in his office and the day of surgery. After the surgery has been completed and the patient has recovered fully from the anaesthetic, he is allowed to go home. When he is at home, he may be seen by a nurse, or arrangements may be made for him to be examined by the surgeon in his office. At that time, the dressing may be changed and any drains or sutures may be removed. The rationale for all of this is to keep the patient out of hospital, thereby saving the government a good deal of money.

If the patients have been carefully selected by the surgeon, this works very well. Where the system fails is when surgery is done in Day Surgery on a patient who has a serious condition for which he should have been admitted to hospital, or where the home care has not been carried out properly. In some cases the patient does not receive proper care at home because the government has reduced the amount of funds required for home care.

Family doctors are seeing patients today for conditions that were not seen by me when I was doing general practice. They are seeing patients who are **ADDICTED TO DRUGS** such as cocaine, heroin, morphine, amphetamines and many other substances. They are seeing young children who have been sniffing gasoline fumes, glue and many other hallucinogenic substances. They are seeing newborn infants who are going through a period of withdrawal from drugs which have been taken by the mother during her pregnancy.

Dealing with such patients is extremely stressful. It also complicates the diagnosis and treatment of other illnesses and injuries. Besides having to suffer physical and verbal abuse from sometimes unruly patients, the doctors and nurses must always protect themselves so that they do not accidentally contract a serious infection while treating these patients. Wearing sterile gloves has become standard procedure when taking blood samples, examining wounds and doing minor surgery. An accidental puncture by a contaminated needle could prove to be fatal. This has changed the whole attitude towards the treatment of emergencies.

Young doctors find it unbelievable when I tell them that I am not aware of seeing a single addict during my years of general practice. When I broached this subject with Dr. Appleby, he reminded me of the one and only addict with which he had to deal. This fellow was travelling from Prince George to Vancouver, appeared at the emergency room, and masqueraded as a patient who had severe abdominal pain due to a recurrence of malaria. When Dr. Appleby saw the patient, his abdomen was extremely tender and rigid on examination. He was admitted to hospital for observation and treatment. After forty-eight hours, it became apparent that this patient was requiring an inordinate amount of morphine in order to control the pain.

Suspecting that things did not add up, Dr. Appleby examined the patient's abdomen after giving him intravenous pentothal. There was no rigidity and no enlargement of the liver. When the patient awakened, Dr. Appleby confronted him and he admitted to being a narcotic addict. He was reported to the RCMP and discharged from hospital. That was Dr. Appleby's one and only experience with narcotic addiction.

There's a follow-up to the above story. Several weeks after Dr. Appleby had discharged the addict from hospital, a young couple appeared in Dr.

Appleby's office one afternoon. They admitted to being drug addicts and said they were on their way to Vancouver in order to go on the methadone program. They asked Dr. Appleby if he would give them each a shot of morphine to tide them over until they reached Vancouver. He refused to give them any medication and they left the office peacefully. Years later, Dr. Appleby learned that this couple were actually R.C.M.P. officers. They had purposely dropped into his office to request a "shot" because the word had been spread around Prince George by the addicts that there was a doctor in Quesnel (Appleby) who was a "soft touch". Apparently the local R.C.M.P. in Quesnel had failed to notify the other R.C.M.P. detachments in the province that Dr. Appleby had realized that his patient was an addict, had discharged him from hospital and had reported him to the R.C.M.P.

Many addicts become very adept at mimicking conditions which cause severe pain, such as gallstones, kidney stones, acute appendicitis and perforated peptic ulcer. If they succeed in fooling an unsuspecting doctor, they are able to get a free ride on morphine for a few hours or longer.

When we see what is happening today all over Canada, but especially in cities such as Vancouver, Toronto and Montreal, it is difficult to believe that I did not see one patient who was addicted to narcotics, stimulants, hallucinogenics, nor any of the numerous drugs that are in common use today. At that time there were only two substances to which people were commonly addicted, alcohol and tobacco. Needless to say, there were a number of alcoholics in our community as there are in every village and town. Of course the doctors were well aware of who they were as we had taken our turns being called to see them (usually in the middle of the night) for minor injuries, illnesses and family problems associated with the excess use of ethanol.

It did not take me long to realize that alcoholism was a self-inflicted condition and that the only person who is able to control the problem (there is no cure) is the patient himself. I did not attempt lecturing the alcoholic on his problem but always advised him to give some serious consideration to joining Alcoholics Anonymous. This still remains the salvation for most of these people.

In the 1970s, a condition known as Fetal Alcohol Syndrome was described. The syndrome affected the infants of women who had ingested alcohol during their pregnancy. The condition consists of mental retardation, failure to grow normally, small skull size, short-sightedness, facial abnormalities, cardiac defects, and abnormalities of the limbs and joints. Since the severity of the defects is directly related to the amount of alcohol consumed daily by the woman during the pregnancy, it is recommended that alcoholic beverages be eliminated completely from the diet. Since there is no treatment for this condition, the objective is prevention.

CONTRACEPTION was, and continues to be, an important component of general practice. Natural family planning methods depend on predicting the time of ovulation by use of basal body temperature or assessment of cervical mucus. This was used by many women in the 1950s, mainly because of the religious ban on contraception.

The most common method of contraception for an unmarried woman consisted in having her partner use a condom. The majority of married women used a vaginal diaphragm which had been fitted accurately by her doctor. A spermicidal jelly was also applied to the side of the diaphragm which came into contact with the cervix. The use of various types of intra-uterine devices (I.U.D.s) is a highly effective method of preventing pregnancy. However, complications such as uterine perforation, excessive bleeding and infection dissuaded many women from using this method of contraception.

Until the Criminal Code was amended, sterilization of the male by vasectomy or the female by tubal ligation, was prohibited. Vasectomy is a simple surgical procedure which can be carried out under local anaesthesia. Tubal ligation can be carried out using the laparoscope, thus avoiding an incision or by laparotomy (opening the abdomen). At the present time, these two procedures are not only legal, but can be performed in such a manner that they are reversible should the person have a change of heart at a later date.

Of course, one of the most dramatic events of the twentieth century was the discovery of the use of steroids in the prevention of conception. The combined estrogen-progestin preparations have proven to be the most effective method of contraception. Simply labelled *The Pill,* it has become the most popular and most effective of all the contraceptives (with the exception of sterilization of course).

Although **SMOKING** has been popular for centuries, it was not until recently that scientists began to study its effects on health. By the 1940s, it had been shown that smoking was the major cause of cancer of the larynx and lungs. Scientists have also shown that smoking is a contributing cause of chronic bronchitis, emphysema and heart disease.

I saw many patients with hoarseness and chronic productive cough due to excessive smoking. I recall one man in particular (not a patient of mine) who requested that I give him a "shot" of penicillin for his cough. He told me that this was the way his doctor usually treated him. He was a very heavy smoker. He was not very happy when I told him that penicillin was not the answer to his problem, but that he should stop smoking. He never did take that advice. In the early 1980s, I heard that he had developed terminal bronchogenic carcinoma (lung cancer). He died soon after. Today, more and more people are giving up cigarettes – except for one group. The number of teenage girls who are smoking is still continuing to rise. They still believe that smoking is the "in thing".

In the 1950s, the **THREAT OF BEING SUED** by a patient was a very low risk for a doctor who was practising good medicine. Not once did a patient threaten to sue me or my associates. At that time, for a lawsuit to be successful, it was necessary for the patient to prove that the doctor had been "negligent". We made mistakes, as everyone did, but that was not considered to be just cause for being found negligent. We missed diagnoses, as every doctor did at times. No one can be right all of the time. Again, that was not considered negligence.

When the law changed and it became possible to successfully sue a doctor for matters such as lack of informed consent, missed diagnoses, complications of surgery, failure to obtain perfect results and dissatisfaction of results by the patient, then the number of lawsuits began to escalate. The adoption of contingency fee billing by the legal profession added to the increase of litigation. The damages awarded by judges and/or juries went from hundreds or thousands of dollars to millions. The cost of malpractice insurance provided by the Canadian Medical Protective Association (which is in essence a "self-insured" program available to properly licenced physicians practicing in Canada) went from twenty-five dollars per year in 1951 to thousands of dollars per year, per doctor, in the 1990s (depending on the area of medicine involved).

As a result, doctors began to practice "defensive medicine". They became concerned more about how to minimize the risk of being successfully sued than focusing entirely on providing what was the best treatment for the patient. Innumerable laboratory tests, x-rays, CAT scans and other expensive investigative procedures were ordered in order to "cover all of the bases" - just in case they might happen to be sued at a later date. Lawsuits were now being brought for "acts of omission" as well as "acts of commission".

The net effect has been to increase the cost of medical care by a disconcertingly alarming amount. Today, it is often the surgeons who are at the forefront of treatment, who are handling the most difficult of cases, who are most likely to be sued. However, no doctor is immune from being faced with litigation.

In spite of the fact that I was never sued, there are two instances I can recall which made me think of the possibility of being sued. The first of these involved a child on whom I had removed the tonsils and adenoids. After transferring the patient to the recovery room, I made my hospital rounds to check on my patients. When I had finished seeing the patients, I returned to the recovery room to check on my patient, before going to the office. As I looked at this young girl, I noticed that there was a tiny blister on each cheek.

At first I was puzzled as to what might have been the cause of these blisters. However, it did not take me long to figure out the most likely reason. While we are doing this type of surgery, it is customary to place a special mouth gag into the patient's mouth in order to keep the mouth wide open. The mouth gag is made of stainless steel.

To prevent damaging the patient's teeth, the part of the gag which fits between the teeth is covered with a rubber tubing. However, the part of the gag where the hinges are located is not covered with the tubing and therefore comes into contact with the cheeks of the patient. At that time, the instruments were sterilized prior to surgery by the use of steam. They were therefore very hot when they were removed from the sterilizer. The instruments were then placed into a basin of cold, sterile water in order to cool them prior to their use. I reasoned that the sides of the mouth gag must have been hot when I placed the gag into the patient's mouth and that neither the nurse nor I had noticed this. This was probably due to the insulating effect of our surgical gloves.

In any event, the metal was hot enough to cause second-degree burns of the patient's cheeks. When I explained this to the mother, she accepted this without getting upset. I arranged to see the patient in the office in two weeks in order to check on her condition. At that time the burned areas were completely healed with no scarring. Needless to say, both the mother and I were relieved.

The second incident involved a woman in her mid-forties who had been admitted to hospital for a hysterectomy. She had been having excessively-heavy menstrual periods and a curettage had shown what is known as a Swiss-cheese endometrium. (The endometrium is the lining of the uterus.) This was considered to be a pre-malignant condition. A hysterectomy was therefore recommended. The surgery was carried out in the usual fashion without incident.

However, while the patient was recovering in the hospital, she noticed a clear, amber-coloured discharge coming from the vagina. I examined her carefully, but could find no cause for the discharge. I instilled a dye called methylene blue into the urinary bladder to see if this would be of any help in locating the problem. On inspection of the vagina, following the instillation of the dye, I noticed a tiny opening in the wall of the vagina through which the coloured fluid flowed. It was then quite obvious to me that the patient had a small communication between the urinary bladder and the vagina – a vesicovaginal fistula. What had obviously occurred was that in putting in the sutures after removing the uterus, one of the sutures had inadvertently penetrated the wall of the bladder. This caused a small area of tissue to break down resulting in the fistula.

Closure of the fistula required another minor surgical procedure. This was carried out immediately and healing occurred without further incident. Of course the patient was not happy when I had informed her of the problem and that another surgical procedure would be required. However, her disappointment was mitigated somewhat when we got the pathologist's report a few days later. An early cancer of the cervix had been identified. Since there had been no sign of this prior to the surgery, she was thankful that the cancer had been detected at such an early stage. Again, this patient did not even hint at the possibility of suing me for the complication.

I believe there were a number of reasons why I was not threatened with a lawsuit for these surgical complications. At that time, in Canada, patients were not as litigation-conscious as they were in the United States. They had not reached the point where they were looking for someone to blame every time things did not turn out as expected. The fact that I did not try to hide my mistakes from the patients, but informed them honestly of what had happened helped me to retain the good rapport I had with them. They trusted me and were willing to accept the fact that I had made an honest mistake. They did not think I had been careless nor negligent. As well, the legal profession in Canada had not yet followed the American way of contingency fee billing, advertising and ambulance chasing.

When the various law societies in Canada changed the rules and legalized such things, the number of law suits began to escalate. A day doesn't go by now when an advertisement by a law firm does not appear on television. The yellow pages of the telephone directories are filled with ads by lawyers and law firms. People are encouraged to seek legal action for anything and everything. The possibility of monetary gain appears to be more important to many patients now than retaining a healthy doctor-patient relationship.

A serious problem being faced by today's practitioners is **CHILD ABUSE** in its many forms.

Doctors caring for emergencies must forever remind themselves that these "accidents" might have been inflicted by a parent or guardian. Reports of such incidents did not appear in the medical literature until the 1960s when authors talked about the so-called "battered child syndrome". Gradually the term used for these non-accidental injuries was "child-abuse". Child abuse included many things other than purely physical injury. Sexual abuse, physical neglect, emotional trauma, lack of proper nourishment, shelter and clothing, and failure to seek proper medical care were found to be common occurrences.

Physical abuse appears in many forms and degrees: abrasion of the skin, slap marks, bruises, burns of various parts of the body, fractures and dislocations, abdominal injuries with damage to the bowel, liver and spleen and skull fractures with damage to the brain. Some of these injuries are severe enough to result in permanent disability or even death. It was stressed that doctors should be alerted to the possibility of non-accidental injuries by answering questions such as the following: is the injury in keeping with the developmental capacity of the infant or child? is the history offered by the parent consistent with the clinical findings? was there an unusual delay in seeking medical attention?

Certain injuries were more likely to arouse suspicion of abuse: immersion burns involving the buttocks and lower extremities, bruises in various stages of healing, multiple rib fractures, multiple fractures in various stages of healing and scarring from previous injuries. It has been estimated that as many as ten percent of injured children seen in emergency rooms of hospitals have been subjected to abuse.

What are the reasons for the plethora of non-accidental injuries? Is it related to the widespread use of drugs? Are young mothers who are single finding it impossible to cope with the care of an infant or young child? Is there a decrease in morality and respect for life? Is there a loss of perception between right and wrong? Have the courts been too lenient when sentencing abusers of children? Are we too willing to return abused children to the care of the abusers? Have we really taken these heinous acts seriously enough?

Far be it from me to suggest that such things did not exist in the 1950s and 1960s. Human nature has not changed since the sins of our first parents. However, I doubt if there are many who `would disagree that child abuse has become a common and serious problem in present-day society. Try as I have, I cannot think of a single instance when I saw a child whom I suspected had been abused by his parents. Was this because I had not been alerted to the possibility by my teachers? Was it because I could not imagine a parent being that sadistic? Was I that naive? Practising in a small community, knowing most of the families and their living conditions intimately, I was in an ideal position to be aware of their social and economic problems. I find it difficult to believe that such behavior would have gone unnoticed.

In 1954, I became a member of the College of General Practice. This organization had been formed in 1953 for the purpose of encouraging general practitioners to embark on a program of *CONTINUING EDUCATION*. There were specific educational requirements which had to be completed in order to become a member, and a certain number of hours of courses required every two years in order to retain the membership. Since I had just completed a full year of training in obstetrics, I was eligible for membership.

It wasn't long after I became a member that I was asked if I would consider taking on a preceptorship. This would entail having a fourth-year medical student from U.B.C. come to Quesnel and spend two weeks with me and my family. Although it would interfere considerably with my regular schedule, I agreed to do it. The student lived with me and my family, slept in the bedroom in the basement, ate his meals with us, accompanied me to the office, went with me when I made house calls, followed me to the emergency room and delivery room, and was by my side whenever I did surgery or gave an anaesthetic. He was my shadow for two weeks.

Both of us learned quite a bit during that period. He learned what it was like to conduct a country practice. I learned what was being taught to medical students at that time. It was a very enjoyable time for the both of us. We were able to discuss many of the problems faced by the doctor who practises in a small town remote from the facilities and the specialists who are readily available in the larger centres. The country doctor must learn quickly to rely on his own judgment as to whether he has the knowledge, courage and skill to manage the patient, or to refer him to the appropriate specialist. Fortunately, most of them do learn this. Some of them never do.

.   One afternoon, while the student was with me in the office, a young mother and her daughter of six years of age came in to see me. The reason for bringing her in to see me was that she had noticed that the girl had recently become quite nervous, was having difficulty sleeping and seemed to be losing weight in spite of the fact that she had a very good appetite. The findings on examining this young patient were quite striking. Her skin was warm and moist. I was shocked to find that her heart rate was one hundred and forty. She had a slight tremor of her fingers. The thyroid gland was enlarged, soft and non-tender. These findings were in keeping with a toxic goitre, also known as hyperthyroidism with enlargement of the thyroid gland. This condition is not unusual in adults, but is very rarely seen in a person six years of age.

I advised the mother of the problem and recommended referral to Vancouver for treatment. I phoned Dr. Ying Chou, a paediatrician, and arranged to have him see her. She was treated medically with a new preparation called propylthiouracil. She responded dramatically to this medication and within a short time returned to her normal self. I have always been amazed that her heart was able to withstand the severe strain put upon it by the overactive thyroid gland. Without proper treatment, she probably would have developed heart failure.

Fifty years ago, the only *SEXUALLY TRANSMITTED DISEASES* of any significance were gonorrhea and syphilis. Today, the list includes chlamydia, genital herpes, chancroid, hepatitis B, Human papillomavirus and the Human Immunodeficiency Virus, which causes Acquired Immune Deficiency Syndrome, more commonly referred to as AIDS. In 1980, AIDS was unknown to medical science. Today, it is an increasing cause of death among young adults in the United States.

In the late 1970s, physicians on the East and the West coasts of the United States began caring for patients who presented with complications of severe immune deficiency, but in whom a known cause of immune suppression could not be identified. These patients, sexually active homosexual men, presented with conditions such as Kaposi's Sarcoma, Pneumocystis carinii pneumonia, oral and esophageal candidiasis and other infections characteristic of severely depressed, cell-mediated immunity. Soon afterwards, similar complications were noted among intravenous drug users, and subsequently among recipients of transfused blood and blood products, including patients with hemophilia. This disease was subsequently called Acquired Immune Deficiency

Syndrome (AIDS). It was found to be caused by a newly-identified virus named human immunodeficiency virus (HIV).

This virus infects the T-helper lymphocytes, leading over a period of years to the depletion of these cells and the development of progressive, severe, irreversible immune deficiency. Over the years, infection with this virus has spread throughout the world and has produced a pandemic of AIDS.

There are now 40 million people infected with HIV/AIDS around the globe. Canada's HIV/AIDS infection rate is 0.3 per cent. The majority of HIV-infected individuals are asymptomatic and are undiagnosed serologically. The virus is transmitted by sexual intercourse, sharing of needles by intravenous drug users, and during pregnancy and delivery of infected women. The virus may be present in the blood, genital secretions, seminal fluid and breast milk. It may also be transmitted via transfused blood.

There are really only two ways for an adult to avoid contracting this fatal illness. The first is to refrain from sexual contact with any person who might harbor the infection. How can you be absolutely sure of this? The partner would have to be tested properly beforehand to be sure he is free of infection. Then a strictly monogamous relationship would have to be adhered to. Can this be guaranteed in these days of complete sexual freedom?

The second preventative would be for intravenous drug users to use a new sterile needle every time they inject themselves. Is this likely to occur? I wouldn't want to bet my life on it. The only absolute guarantee of freedom from being infected is total abstinence, which appears to be out of the question for most people. They appear to believe that the reward is worth the risk.

In spite of what "experts" and "educators" might be preaching, there is no such thing as "safe sex" when it comes to AIDS. The use of condoms, which has been widely proclaimed as the method of choice in prophylaxis against AIDS, is no guarantee in preventing transmission of this disease. There is always the possibility that the virus may be transmitted to a partner through slippage of the condom, passage through a break in the latex, improper application, and even a defect during the manufacturing process. When one stops to consider that there is no cure for this condition, and that it is invariably fatal, is it worth taking the risk? In my opinion, only a fool would do so.

This subject reminds me of two events which occurred when I was in my fourth and final year of medical school. At the time, I didn't consider them to be major events, but when I reflect on them now, they were unusual. The first event occurred one Saturday morning when the head of the department of obstetrics and gynecology walked into the classroom. As he stood in the front of the class, he reached into his pocket and pulled out a condom which had been removed previously from its package.

He then proceeded to unroll the condom onto his left index and middle fingers. He informed us that this was the proper method of applying a condom for contraceptive purposes. He then rolled the condom up and put it back into his pocket. He then proceeded to discuss some other subject which was neither related to contraception nor to his specialty. This was the one and only time that contraceptive technique was described to my class by anyone during my four years of medical school. Unbelievable? I can hardly believe it myself, but it is a fact.

The second event was a little more surprising to the class, but lasted for even a shorter period of time than the previous one. One of our instructors in psychiatry used to come to the medical school at times from the mental hospital at Ponoka, where he was a staff member. On this particular afternoon, he was to give the first lecture after our lunch break. He walked into the classroom, stood at the front of the class, looked around the class for about ten seconds, and then brought everyone to attention by saying "*It is generally considered that about one in every thirty people is homosexual*".

Since there were thirty-six students in the class, every one of us immediately scanned each and every other member expecting, I suppose, to be able to pick out the unfortunate statistic. Of course, no one seemed to be guilty. The words gay and lesbian were not used in those days, at least in my circle of acquaintances. As a matter of fact, even the word homosexual was used only during jokes on the subject, which were rare. It seemed that the subject not considered to be important.

To our surprise, and perhaps relief, he did not lecture on the subject of homosexuality as one might have expected him to do. Instead, he proceeded to discuss some other psychiatric condition that wasn't remotely related to sex. Why he had even mentioned the subject in the manner he did remains a mystery to me. I can't recall having a single lecture on the subject of homosexuality during the four years of medical school. Unbelievable? We didn't seem to be upset by not being taught anything about a fairly common condition.

It was many years later that I would learn that there was in fact one member of our class who was homosexual. If any other members of the class were aware of this, it was certainly a well-kept secret. This classmate was a quiet person, polite, and exhibited no unusual behavior characteristics. He was a good student, and became a very good neurologist. The last time I saw him was during a class reunion held in Vancouver in the early 1980s. At the time he appeared to be perfectly healthy. However, not many months were to pass before I heard that he had died. Cause of death? AIDS.

The only *EATING PROBLEM* encountered by me while in general practice was one which was, and continues to be, the most common one, namely obesity. This is affecting more and more people due to the change in our eating habits and the decrease in physical activity. People who are overweight refuse message that excess weight is simply due ~~~ that they are consuming more calories ~ utilizing. They do not believe that ...g one's weight and retaining the weight reduction requires a change in lifestyle. They are still hoping for some magic formula. Instead of reducing their intake of high-calorie foods and increasing the amount of daily exercise, they hope to have a rapid drop in weight by going on one of the various popular diets. The fact that the shelves of bookstores are replete with dozens and dozens of books advocating various guaranteed diets should be enough to convince them that this is the wrong approach to the problem.

There are two specific eating problems which have been with us for centuries. They have become extremely common in the past twenty years. I'm referring to anorexia nervosa and bulimia. Although I did not encounter any patients with these conditions, I'm sure family doctors are seeing many patients with these conditions today. They represent a real challenge to today's practitioners.

Anorexia nervosa is a syndrome in which caloric intake insufficient to maintain one's weight is associated with a delusion of being fat. There is an obsession to be thinner. Patients with anorexia nervosa believe they are fat, even when they are emaciated. They are driven to lose more and more weight by vomiting, dieting, exercising and using cathartics. True anorexia nervosa is not present until there has been extreme weight loss. Anorexia nervosa is a very serious eating disorder with a mortality rate of around 10%. The patient with this condition should be under the care of a medical practitioner who specializes in eating disorders.

Bulimia is an eating disorder in which there are recurrent episodes of binge eating. Binge eating refers to the rapid consumption of large amounts of food over a short period of time, usually less than two hours. During the eating episodes, there is the fear of not being able to stop the eating. The gorging is followed by self-induced vomiting. The person also resorts to excessive exercise, misuse of laxatives, diuretics, enemas and other medications. Since the person is aware of her eating problem, there is an associated depression along with self-deprecating thoughts.

The development of *NEW DRUGS* has had a profound effect on the ability of the family doctor to treat his patients. The first important step was the discovery of chemotherapeutic agents which could be used to treat infections. Although the sulfa drug sulfanilamide was discovered in 1908, it was not until 1933 that another sulfa drug, prontosil, was used for the first time in the treatment of a patient. The drug was given to a ten-month-old infant with staphylococcal septicemia. The effect was a dramatic cure.

In 1928, Alexander Fleming accidentally discovered a mold which caused destruction of staphylococcus bacteria on a culture plate. Because the mold belonged to the genus Penicillium, Fleming named the antibacterial substance penicillin. In 1941, penicillin was used experimentally for the first time to treat infections in humans. In 1943, syphilis was treated successfully for the first time with penicillin. Prior to this, syphilis had been incurable.

In the 1950s, sulfa drugs, penicillin and two or three other antibiotics were the mainstay in the treatment of infections. Initially, penicillin had to be given to the patient intramuscularly. My medical bag (which I carried on house calls) contained ampoules of penicillin along with a special syringe with which to administer the drug to the patient. It was a wonderful break-through when penicillin became available in tablet and liquid preparations.

When the antibiotic chloramphenicol became available, it was welcomed with open arms. The liquid preparation was used extensively to treat infections in infants and young children. However, it wasn't long before a serious complication of this drug was reported. A small percentage of patients who had used the drug subsequently developed aplastic anemia. Aplastic anemia is a fatal condition due to depression of the bone marrow (the place where blood cells are formed).

Today, there are dozens of antibiotics available to the practising physician. These new chemotherapeutic agents are not only useful in combating bacterial infections, but also other organisms which cause infections. Some are even effective against viruses.

In 1680, Thomas Sydenham, one of the outstanding physicians of the 17th century, wrote "Among the remedies which it has pleased Almighty God to give to man to relieve his sufferings, none is so universal and so efficacious as Opium". Today, morphine, the alkaloid that gives Opium its analgesic actions, remains the standard against which new analgesics are measured. Many of the newer analgesics may be considered its equal, but it is doubtful that any of them is clinically superior.

Although there is a great deal of controversy today concerning the use of marijuana as an analgesic, the reader might be surprised to learn that in the 1950s it was not unusual for the pharmacist to receive a prescription from a physician for opium. The preparation used at that time was tincture opii (also referred to as paregoric). This preparation was highly effective for two conditions: it was occasionally used to relieve colic in newborn infants and was efficacious in controlling severe diarrhea in adults. The reader might also be surprised to learn that another narcotic which has a bad reputation today because of its non-medical use by addicts, was routinely used by some obstetricians in the 1940s and 1950s for the relief of pain during the early stage of labor. I am referring to heroin, which had a very calming effect on the anxious and tense primigravida.

In the 1950s, we used aspirin and codeine for the relief of mild pain and morphine or demerol for moderate to severe pain. The only real improvement occurred when acetaminophen (tylenol) became available. Since it was available in liquid form, it was much easier to administer to infants and young children. Non-steroidal anti-inflammatory drugs were not available at that time.

Medications for the treatment of emotional and psychiatric problems were practically non-existent. Phenobarbital was used as a mild sedative for the anxious patient and the person who was under a lot of stress. The patient suffering from insomnia was given chloral hydrate, seconal or amytal. When meprobamate (equanil) became available, this was thought to be the "cure-all" for anxiety, stress and panic attacks. Chlordiazepoxide (librium) also proved to be of some benefit for the anxious patient, but it would be some time before tranquilizers were discovered.

The only treatment available for depression was electro-convulsive therapy (electro-shock) or insulin in increasing doses until a state of coma was induced. There were no anti-depressants and the efficacy of lithium for manic-depressive psychosis (bipolar disease) had not been discovered. There was really no specific treatment for major psychoses such as schizophrenia. Anti-psychotic drugs are relatively new.

For many years, psychoanalysis was considered to be "the treatment" for the neurotic patient, but its status has followed that of the dodo bird.

The treatment of cardio-vascular diseases was limited. Nitroglycerin tablets placed under the tongue were used to relieve the angina (chest pain) of the patient suffering from coronary artery disease. It would be a number of years before long-acting nitrate tablets, sublingual sprays and dermal patches would be available. Myocardial infarction (heart attacks) were treated with strict bed rest for several days along with the anti-coagulants heparin and dicumarol.

The use of anti-thrombotic (anti-clot) medications and a continuous intravenous drip of nitroglycerine represent more recent improvements in therapy. Numerous new medications, such as drugs to lower the amount of cholesterol in the blood, beta-blockers and anti-hypertensive agents, have dramatically reduced the death rate from heart disease and strokes. The finding that a small amount of aspirin taken daily will reduce the incidence of heart attacks and strokes was a major therapeutic event.

Of course, no one ever dreamed of open-heart surgery to open coronary arteries, repair holes in the partitions of the heart, replace valves and ultimately to replace the heart itself. The replacement of large arteries with plastic tubes was also a miracle which was yet to occur.

There have been many improvements in the treatment of diabetes since the discovery of insulin by Banting and Best in 1921. We managed our diabetic patients by means of special diets and two types of insulin. Regular insulin acted quickly and lasted for a short period of time. Protamine zinc insulin was slower to act but its effect lasted for a longer period of time. At the present time, there are not only several types of insulin available but also medications which can be taken orally and have the effect of lowering the level of glucose in the blood.

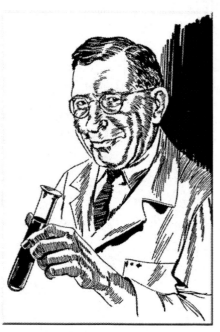

PHOTO 51 [Drawing of Dr. Frederick Banting, one of the Canadian researchers who discovered insulin]

Recent experimental work carried out at the University of Alberta (my Alma Mater) has made possible the transplantation of islet cells (which produce insulin) from the pancreas of one person into a diabetic individual. If it becomes possible to perfect this procedure, the final solution to diabetes will have been found.

Among the achievements the 20th century will be remembered for is the discovery of Vitamins. For hundreds of years people had noticed that some foods seemed to prevent some diseases. The most famous example is the limes and lemons that British sailors ate to prevent scurvy. In 1911, the first Vitamin to be isolated in the laboratory was thiamine, also known as Vitamin B1. Since then, a total of thirteen Vitamins have been discovered.

Vitamins are organic substances that the body requires to help regulate metabolic functions within cells. They are absolutely essential to life. While Vitamins themselves do not supply energy, some do aid in the efficient conversion of foods into energy. Since Vitamins are not manufactured in the body, they must be furnished from an external source. As a general rule, a healthy individual ingesting a well-balanced diet receives adequate amounts of Vitamins from his foods.

When I was in general practice, I recommended the use of Vitamins for three specific classes of patients. It was generally agreed that during pregnancy a woman should take one multi-vitamin tablet daily throughout her pregnancy. The newborn infant was also put on multi-vitamin drops daily for the first year of his life. The third class of patient was the one who had pernicious anemia. This type of anemia is treated with intramuscular injections of Vitamin B12. Since there is no cure for this condition (hence the name pernicious), monthly injections are necessary for as long as the patient lives.

Today, folacin (folic acid) is given to women who are planning to become pregnant. This Vitamin has been found to reduce the incidence of certain birth defects, such as neural tube defects (defects of the vertebrae and spinal cord) in new born infants. In some centres it has become standard procedure to give a single intramuscular dose of Vitamin K to all newborn infants. This has been found to reduce the incidence of spontaneous hemorrhages caused by deficiencies in the blood of substances which are necessary for coagulation. Some nutritional experts recommend that supplements of Vitamin C and Vitamin E be taken daily. They believe that these supplements are safe and that they reduce the risk of heart disease. However, there is still no consensus of opinion concerning these Vitamins.

There is probably no single class of drugs which has been the target of as much quackery, misunderstanding, misrepresentation and misuse as Vitamins. Before embarking on a program of Vitamin supplements, a person would be wise to consult with his family doctor.

Periodically, there is someone who complains that the medical doctor is interested only in the *"treatment" of diseases* and cares little about the *"prevention" of illnesses, injuries and the promotion of good health.* We are portrayed as healers who have been taught very little about keeping the body healthy. Whenever I hear such nonsense, I become upset. In every disease that we studied in medical school, we always learned how the disease could be prevented as well as how it could be treated.

Anyone who doubts that members of the medical profession are not concerned with the prevention of illnesses need only be reminded of the following measures promoted by this profession: Inoculations and Vaccinations for the prevention of infectious diseases, routine serology testing for syphilis in every pregnant woman, Pap. Smears for the early detection of cancer of the cervix, breast self examination following every shower or tub bath, professional breast examination annually for women over 40, mammograms for all women over age 35 and annually after age 50, yearly examination of the prostate and PSA testing as indicated, examination of the testicles accompanying every bath or shower for possible tumors, regular measurement of blood pressure, cholesterol screening, glaucoma screening for everyone over age 65, colon screening for cancer for everyone over age 50 with a family history of cancer of the colon, for anyone with inflammatory bowel disease or polyps in the large intestine, and genetic testing for certain specific conditions.

Medical doctors have also supported anti-smoking campaigns, Mothers Against Drunk Drivers, mandatory seat-belt legislation, mandatory helmets for motorcycles and bicycles, skate boards and hockey, improved nutrition, exercise programs, reduction of exposure to noise in industry and many other programs designed to improve the health of Canadians.

However, even the decision on how to make one's living in the medical profession has become more difficult. Because of the increasing amount of knowledge and the complexities of medicine today, the hospital training of the family doctor is no longer limited to a single year of internship after graduating from medical school. When the medical student has completed his second year of schooling, he is obliged to declare whether he is intending to pursue a career in *FAMILY PRACTICE*, or to proceed into *ONE OF THE SPECIALTIES*.

If he decides that he wishes to be a general practitioner, he will complete the third and fourth years of medical school and then embark on a three-year hospital program designed specifically for the training of family doctors. If he decides that he wishes to be a specialist, he will complete the third and fourth years of medical school and then embark on a four-year residency program in the specialty of his choice. Once he has made the decision at the end of his second year of medical school, there is no turning back.

I believe this has been a foolish decision by the faculties of the medical schools and the doctors in charge of the hospital training programs. I make this judgment call for a number of reasons. There are very few medical students who know what type of work they wish to do when they have completed the second year of medical school.

But what is even more important, the student has no idea what he is suited for until he has had considerable exposure to clinical practice. For example, the student may decide that he wishes to be an orthopaedic surgeon, but after being in the residency program for a year or two he may find that he is not only unsuited to that type of work, but that he doesn't even enjoy it. What is he to do, complete the program and become a very unhappy or incapable orthopaedic surgeon? It doesn't make any sense. If the student decides to take the general practice program, completes this, does general practice for three or four years and then decides that he would prefer to be an obstetrician, he is out of luck. There is no way he will be accepted into a residency program because the programs are already filled. Many of the best specialists are those who have done general practice for a number of years and then have gone on to become specialists. This is no longer possible.

In view of this, I suspect there will be a high percentage of students who will become specialists because they do not want to take the risk of being locked into general practice once they have made this decision. This is unfortunate when there is such a tremendous need for family doctors.

There is an urgent need for family doctors in the cities, towns and villages of this country. More must be done to encourage young men and women to consider spending at least a portion of their medical careers in such a worthwhile, satisfying and spiritually rewarding career. The general practitioners in the rural areas of British Columbia are still doing a good deal of surgery, obstetrics and anaesthesia. Although many of the smaller cities are fortunate now to have specialists such as general surgeons and internists, there is still much work left to be done by the family doctor.

Canadian doctors who graduated since the 1970s have no idea what it was like to practice medicine prior to *MEDICARE*. My experience in general practice was unique not only in that it was country practice in a relatively isolated community, but also because it spanned a ten-year period prior to Medicare. Before the introduction of medicare, patients were personally responsible for payment of their medical bills. Although there were some private medical insurers such as Medical Services Association, , C.U. and C. and Fraser Valley Medical, most of the people living in the Cariboo did not have any medical insurance. They were totally responsible for the payment of the doctor's bill and also the hospital bill.

The doctor's fees were set by the B.C. Medical Association. The Association published a booklet known as the Minimum Schedule of Fees. This booklet was distributed to every doctor practising in British Columbia. It listed various items such as office visit, house call, maternity care, various surgical procedures, and so on, and the appropriate fee for these services. For example, in 1951, the fee for an office visit was $5.00, that for a house call was $6.00, the maternity fee was $50.00 and the fee for the removal of tonsils and adenoids was $30.00. The fee for seeing a Native from the reserve in the Nazko Valley was $1.00. This was paid by the federal government. If the fee was not submitted by the proper date, it was not paid.

All of this changed with the onset of Medicare. Doctors are now paid for almost 100% of their billings by the provincial and federal governments.

Canada's national health insurance program is designed to ensure that every resident of Canada receives medical care. The cost of this care is paid through general taxes and health-insurance premiums.

In 1957, the federal government passed the Hospital Insurance and Diagnostic Act. This Act gave the federal government authority to enter into an agreement with the provinces to establish a comprehensive, universal plan covering acute hospital care, laboratory and radiology services. In 1962, Medicare had its beginning in the province of Saskatchewan when Tommy Douglas was Premier. As a result, Douglas is generally considered to be the Father of Medicare. In 1964, the report of Justice Emmett Hall's Royal Commission recommended universal Medicare. By 1972, all provinces and territories had embraced Medicare.

At the onset of Medicare, the federal government agreed to pay 50% of the cost of universal medicare while the other 50% was to be paid by the provinces. However, it did not take long before the federal government began to reduce its share of the cost. At the present time, the federal government is paying less than 20% of the cost.

In 1984, the Canada Health Act was passed by the federal government. The Act was passed to prevent extra-billing and user fees by doctors. The five conditions of this legislation have become the five principles of our health care system. In order to receive transfer of funds from the federal government, the provinces must meet these five specific criteria which are: public administration, comprehensiveness, universality, portability and accessibility.

In 1992, the Provincial/Territorial Conference of Ministers of Health met in Banff, Alberta. At this meeting, the following resolutions were passed:

1.   To reduce by the fall of 1993 Canadian medical school entry class size by 10 percent.

2.   To reduce national postgraduate medical training positions by 10 percent.

3.   To reduce the recruitment of Visa trainee graduates of foreign medical schools into Canada for postgraduate medical training.

The effect of these policies is that we now have a severe shortage of trained physicians and surgeons in every part of Canada. It will take many years before there is an adequate number of doctors in this country.

There are now private labs where patients are able to have CAT scans and MRI tests carried out quickly if they are willing and able to pay the price. Fees for these procedures are paid for by the Workers' Compensation Board.

There are also private clinics where patients are able to have surgery carried out which is not covered by Medicare, such as cosmetic surgery. Workers who are also covered by the Workers' Compensation Board are also encouraged to use these facilities because the surgery can be carried out more quickly, thereby allowing the workman to return to work in a matter of days or weeks rather than months.

Today, there are thousands of people who have no family doctor and are unable to find one. When they become ill, they have two choices; they can go to the emergency room of the hospital, or they can go to a walk – in clinic. Since many of these illnesses are minor, the effect is to clog the emergency rooms. This makes it extremely difficult for the nurses and doctors. If they elect to go to a walk – in clinic, they can be seen within a few minutes. No appointment is needed. Since the clinics are open during the evenings, Saturdays, Sundays and holidays, they serve a genuine purpose especially for working people.

Today, patients have to wait long periods of time in order to be seen by specialists to whom they have been referred. They may then have to wait for days, weeks or even months for diagnostic tests and for surgery. Some patients are unable to receive treatment in their own communities and must be transferred to other hospitals, cities, or provinces. There are a few who must be transferred to the United States for treatment.

CHAPTER 16: TIME TO MOVE ON

Burned Out

Medicine is the most jealous of all mistresses.
Louis Beauchamp, Edmonton Paediatrician

In 1955, Dr. Avery decided that he would like to get more training in surgery. Although he was capable of doing many of the difficult surgical procedures generally reserved for certified general surgeons, and had done so on many occasions, he felt the need for further training. He was fortunate in being able to arrange to take a year of training at St. Paul's Hospital. This was a great sacrifice on his part as it meant that he was able to spend only the occasional weekend with his family who had remained in Quesnel during this period of time. The year of surgery proved to be very valuable to us and the people of Quesnel when he returned. He was quite capable of doing most of the surgical procedures which were required at that time.

I felt that Dr. Avery never received the appreciation which was due to him for the years that he had spent in the Cariboo. When he first arrived in Quesnel in the mid 1940s as a young man, Dr. Baker was the only doctor practising at the time. He joined Dr. Baker and slowly but steadily worked to improve the quality of medical care in the area. Although it is true that Dr. Baker had done a wonderful job working for many years on his own, there is a limit to what one man can do no matter how capable and dedicated he may be.

Dr. Avery organized the Quesnel Clinic and ran it in a more modern fashion. Prior to his coming to Quesnel, patients would walk into the clinic at any time, for any reason, without an appointment. Sometimes this could be chaotic. Dr. Avery insisted that patients arrange appointments for specific times, except for emergencies, which were always tended to immediately. He also made an effort to have patients who could afford to, pay for their care. Some of these changes were not popular with many of the older patients in town who were used to arriving at the office at their convenience and ignoring bills for services. It is much easier to love a doctor and praise him when he doesn't charge you, than it is if he requests fair compensation.

As a result of Dr. Baker's poor business sense, I suspect that after over 40 years of active practice, he died a relatively poor man. This does not represent much of a "thank you" for a job well done. Of course there are many memorials today celebrating the life of Dr. Baker – all acquired after his death.

By 1959, Dr. Avery's older children were reaching the age when they would soon be attending university. In view of this, he made the decision to move to Vancouver. It was not easy to find a replacement for him. However, we were very fortunate in finding a surgeon who was willing to move to Quesnel. Dr. Jack Simpson had just completed a four – year training program in England, had passed the Canadian specialty examinations and was interested in moving to the Cariboo. He had been born and raised in Edmonton and was a graduate of the University of Alberta. After interning in Edmonton, Jack had gone to England where he had acquired excellent training in all areas of general surgery. He was an exceptionally capable surgeon.

I had the privilege of caring for his wife Mary during her first pregnancy and delivered their first son, Christopher.

By 1961, I had become so busy in my practice that I had very little time to spend with my family and almost no time for medical reading or study. I began to get frustrated in not being able to study and keep up with the advances in medicine which related to my type of practice.

The final straw came when I was treating an infant who was three weeks old and had severe gastroenteritis. In spite of doing a cutdown, administering I-V fluids and antibiotics, the infant died. The only saving grace, if you could call it that, was that the baby was the tenth child in the family. In spite of the fact that I had run back and forth from the office to the hospital several times to check on the baby, I couldn't help feeling that if I had cancelled all of my office appointments and spent all of my time at the hospital, things might have turned out differently.

It was then that I made the decision that I would leave general practice and embark on a specialty in which I could have more control over my time. At this time I did not know which specialty I wished to pursue. I needed time away from the hustle and bustle of a very busy practice in order to consider my options.

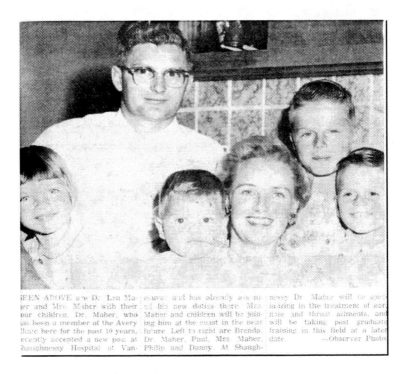

PHOTO 52 [Photo contained in a newspaper clipping taken from the *Cariboo Observer* that depicts the author and his family around the time of moving from Quesnel]

In July of 1951, as a young, energetic, inexperienced doctor, I made the journey from Vancouver to Quesnel with my wife and infant son. I was eager to test the knowledge I had acquired in medical school and internship. In September of 1961, having obtained a wealth of experience in family practice, I departed from the Cariboo with my wife and four young children. I had not yet set my compass, but I knew that whatever course I took I would once more be starting at the bottom of the ladder. It would be a number of years before I would become competent and comfortable in my new career as a specialist.

ABOUT THE AUTHOR

Dr. Maher graduated in 1949 from the University of Alberta with a degree in medicine.

He did a year's rotating internship at St. Paul's Hospital in Vancouver followed by a year in the departments of Medicine and Pediatrics.

In 1951, with his wife and infant son, he travelled to Quesnel to work with Dr. Frank Avery and Dr. Gerald Baker.

In 1953, he returned to Edmonton where he was resident in Obstetrics and Gynecology at the new maternity unit of the Royal Alexandra Hospital.

He returned to Quesnel in 1954 and continued to work at the Avery Clinic until 1961. He left Quesnel in 1961, spent a year in the department of Otolaryngology at Shaughnessy Hospital in Vancouver, and then travelled with his wife and four children to Richmond, Virginia.

After completing a three-year residency in Otolaryngology at the Medical College of Virginia, he returned to Kamloops B.C. where he practised general Otolaryngology until 1975 and Otology until 1985.

Following coronary by-pass surgery in 1985, he retired to Rivershore Golf Course in Kamloops where he resides with his wife.

LIST OF PHOTOGRAPHS AND DIAGRAMS

Cover – Author and two classmates (now both deceased) carrying out dissection of head and neck of their cadaver – First Year Anatomy Class at Medical School

281

ISBN 1-41205926-7

9 781412 059268